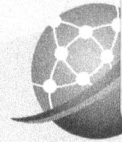

Prep Your Way
Workshops | Online Courses | Workbooks

Associate Safety Professional (ASP)	**Certified Instructional Trainer (CIT)**	**Certified Hazardous Materials Manager (CHMM)**
Construction Health and Safety Technician (CHST)	**Certified Industrial Hygienist (CIH)**	**Certified Safety Professional (CSP)**
Occupational Hygiene and Safety Technologist (OHST)	**Safety Management Specialist (SMS)**	**Safety Trained Supervisor (STS)**

Safety Trained Supervisor Construction (STSC)

SPAN™ **Exam Prep** is the leading certification exam study solution to prepare safety professionals for exams from the Board of Certified Safety Professionals (BCSP). This BCSP exam prep helps professionals achieve important career goals through advancing competencies for safety management excellence. As the leader in BCSP exam preparation since 1992, SPAN offers live workshops, online courses and workbooks. The self-directed study materials are designed for professionals looking to gain critical knowledge, study techniques, and testing strategies to pass certification examinations.

www.spansafety.com

Dedicated to All Safety, Health and Environmental Professionals

Striving to Protect

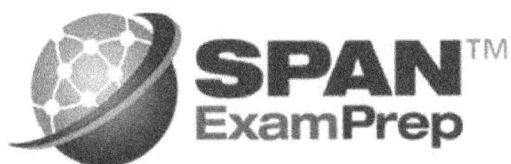

SPAN™ ExamPrep

www.spansafety.com

This Publication may not cover every aspect of the certification process and is not intended as a guarantee that the user will pass an exam or become certified.

The information contained in this study workbook is intended to be used in preparation for the Certified Industrial Hygienist® examination and should not be used as an authority in the professional practice of safety, health, or environmental compliance.

The Certified Industrial Hygienist® (CIH®) Certification is a registered trademark of the American Board of Industrial Hygienists (ABIH).

The opinions expressed are those of the authors and no guarantee, warranty, or other representation is made as to the absolute correctness or sufficiency of any information contained in this study workbook.

Daniel J. Snyder, Ed.D, CSP, CHMM, OHST, CET
Tim C. Sterling, MPH, CIH, CSP, OHST

Copyright © 2019 by SPAN™ International Training, LLC
402 W. Mt Vernon St #111
Nixa, Missouri 65714
Phone: (417) 724-8348
info@spansafetyworkshops.com

ISBN 978-1-886786-37-0 (set)
ISBN 978-1-886786-38-7 (v.1)
ISBN 978-1-886786-39-4 (v.2)

Contents

Rubric 13: Ionizing Radiation

Ionizing radiation is radiation with enough energy to remove electrons from the orbit of an atom, thus causing the atom to become charged or ionized. There are two forms: waves and particles.

Alexander Litvinenko, a former Russian spy, was killed in November 2006. At the time, the 43-year old was secretly working for British intelligence investigating the operations of the Russian mafia in Spain.

Mr. Litvinenko became ill soon after having tea with two other Russian operatives. He spent the night vomiting, and three days later, he was hospitalized in serious condition. He died within three weeks of the onset of symptoms.

Testing and a post-mortem examination identified the cause of death as polonium-210 poisoning.

The investigation led to detecting polonium-210 at the Millennium Hotel, a nightclub, the British embassy in Moscow, two airplanes, and the Emirates stadium.

Polonium-210 is silver-colored metal found in uranium ores. It is one of 25 radioactive isotopes of polonium, and as it decays, alpha particles are emitted. Polonium-210 has a life of 138 days.

Important Terms and Concepts

Absorbed Dose (RAD) – The energy deposited by radiation into a mass of material. RAD is the unit of measure and the acronym for 'Radiation Absorbed Dose.' *Note* 1 Gy = 100 RAD.

Activity (Radioactivity) – The number of decays the radiological material undergoes per unit of time. Historically, Curie (Ci) is the unit of decay, but the Bequerel (Bq) is the SI unit.

Attenuation – The process in which a reduction of intensity of a beam, particle, and/or photon is known, but the energy transfer is unknown.

Bequerel (Bq) – SI unit of intensity and expressed as decay per unit of time. 1Bq = 1dps

Compton Effect - A glancing collision of a gamma-photon with an orbital electron. The gamma-photon gives part of its energy to the electron, thus ejecting the electron from its orbit.

Curie (Ci) – The unit for decay. 1 Ci = 3.7×10^{10} dps

Dose Equivalent (REM) – There is no precise meaning, but it is commonly used to address the amount of biological damage produced by a specific radiation and a given exposure. It is determined by Absorbed Dose (RAD or Gy) x quality factor.

Half-life – The length of time for ½ of a group of radioactive atoms to decay to a stable state.

Linear Energy Transfer – The term in dosimetry used for describing the amount of energy deposited per unit of travel through tissue (keV per micrometer). Protons, neutrons and α particles have much greater LET than gamma or x-ray.

Photoelectric Effect – The ejection of an electron from an inner shell upon absorbing the energy of a photon.

REM – The unit for measuring 'dose equivalent'. rem = (rad)(qf)

Roentgen (R) – Historical unit for measuring the quantity of exposure. It is only defined for the amount of ionization produced in air. Not used in modern terminology.

Specific Activity (SA) – The rate of decay for a given mass. For example, Ci/g or Bq/kg. Ionizing radiation has different characteristics including physical state, charge, and hazard presented.

Characteristics for Common Types of Ionizing Radiation

Type	Composition	Typical Energies	Hazard
Alpha Particle	2 protons & 2 neutrons	4-8 MeV	Internal
Beta Particle	Electron	0.018-3 MeV	Internal & External
Gamma Ray	Electro-magnetic wave	0.01-2 MeV	Internal & External
X-Ray	Electro-magnetic wave	0.01-150 keV	Internal & External
Neutron	Free Neutron	0.025 eV-5MeV	External

Radon is a noble gas that has low solubility. It is usually inhaled and exhaled without effect, unless it decays while in the lung. The first few decays create the lung hazard. Po-218 through Po-214 have short half-lives and can deposit energy into lung tissue. Pb-210 has a long half-life and will likely be removed by physiological processes before decaying.

Radon Decay Progeny and Hazard

Progeny	Half-Life	Decay & Energy
Radon-222	3.8 days	Alpha, 5.48 MeV
Polonium-218	3 minutes	Alpha, 6.0 MeV
Lead-214	27 minutes	Beta
Bismuth-214	20 minutes	Beta
Polonium-214	180 microseconds	Alpha, 7.69 MeV
Lead-210	22 years	Beta

U.S. Nuclear Regulatory Commission: 10 CFR 20; Occupational Dose Limit

Description	Annual Limit
Total Effective Dose Equivalent (TEDE)	5 rem (0.05 Sv)
Deep Dose Equivalent and Committed Dose Equivalent (Summation)	50 rem (0.5 Sv)
Eye Dose Equivalent	15 rem (0.15Sv)
Shallow Dose Equivalent to Skin or Extremities	50 rem (0.5 Sv)
NOTE: The 50 rem limit for skin is to prevent nonstochastic effects. Extremity means hand, elbow, arm below elbow, foot, knee, and leg below the knee.	

Equations

Inverse Square Law

$$\frac{I_1}{I_2} = \left[\frac{d_2}{d_1}\right]^2$$

Where:
I_1 is the intensity level at distance 1
I_2 is the intensity level at distance 2
NOTE: I_1 and I_2 must have same units, as does d_1 and d_2
Use:
Can be used with physical energies such as radiation, sound power, illumination for calculating intensity, distance, or dose given any 3 of the 4 variables.

Example:
The intensity at 1 foot from the source is 3 MeV/cm^2. The door to the room is 15 feet from the source. Calculate the intensity at the plane of the door opening.

Step 1: Rearrange the equation to isolate I_2

$$I_2 = I_1 \left(\frac{d_1}{d_2}\right)^2$$

$$I_2 = 3 MeV \left(\frac{1\ foot}{15\ feet}\right)^2$$

$$I_2 = 0.0133\ \text{MeV}$$

Confirm the concept. Moving away from the source decreases intensity, while moving closer increases intensity.

Radioactive Decay

$$A = A_i \left(0.5^{\left(\frac{t}{T_{1/2}} \right)} \right)$$

Where:
A is the radioactivity remaining after time
A_i is the initial radioactivity
t is the time of interest
$T_{1/2}$ is the half-life for the source material
NOTE: The time units must be same and the activity units must be the same (Ci, Bq).
Use:
Determining the level of activity for a source either initially or after a period of time using the half-life.

Example:
A source has an activity of 100 mCi when received at the research lab at 0800. The half-life of the isotope is 12 days. The researcher plans to start working with the material in exactly 2 weeks at 1200. What will the activity be at this time?

Step 1: Solve for t in days

$$2 \text{ weeks} + 4 \text{ hours} = 14.167 \text{ days}$$

Step 2: Solve for activity (A)

$$A = A_i \left(0.5^{\left(\frac{t}{T1/2} \right)} \right)$$

$$A = 100 \; mCi \left(0.5^{\left(\frac{14.167 \; days}{12 \; days} \right)} \right)$$

$$A = 44.12 \text{ mCi}$$

$$A = A_i e^{\frac{-0.693t}{T_{1/2}}}$$

Where:

A is the radioactivity remaining after time

A_i is the initial radioactivity

t is the time of interest

$T_{1/2}$ is the half-life for the source material

NOTE: The time units must be same and the activity units must be the same (Ci, Bq).

Use:

To calculate activity after a given period of time.

Example:

A source has an activity of 100 mCi when received at the research lab at 0800. The half-life of the isotope is 12 days. The researcher plans to start working with the material in exactly 2 weeks at 1200. What will the activity be at this time?

Step 1: Solve for t in days

$$2 \text{ weeks} + 4 \text{ hours} = 14.167 \text{ days}$$

Step 2: Solve for activity (A)

$$A = A_i e^{\frac{-0.693t}{T_{1/2}}}$$

$$A = 100 mCi e^{\frac{-0.693(14.167)}{12}}$$

$$A = 44.12 \text{ mCi}$$

Activity for A Specific Element

$$A = \frac{0.693}{T_{1/2}} N_i$$

Where:
A is the radioactivity of the element
N_i is the number of atoms of the source material
$T_{1/2}$ is the half-life for the source material
NOTE: The time units must be same and the activity units must be the same (Ci, Bq).
Use:
To calculate the radioactivity of an amount of material when the quantity is given as atoms.

Example:
Calculate the radioactivity for 1 µg of iodine 131 in becquerels. I-131 has a half-life of 8 days.

Step 1: Use Avogadro's number to calculate the number of atoms

$$N = \frac{6.023 \ x \ 10^{23}}{131 \ g} x 10^{-6} g$$

$$N = 4.6 \ x \ 10^{15} \text{ atoms}$$

Step 2: Convert the half-life to seconds
8 days x 86400 seconds/day = 691200 seconds

Step 3: Calculate the activity (A) in dps or becquerels

$$A = \frac{0.693}{T_{1/2}} N_i$$

$$A = \frac{0.693}{691200} x (4.6 \ x \ 10^{15})$$

$$A = 4.61 \ x \ 10^9 \text{ dps or becquerel}$$

$$I = \left(\frac{1}{2}\right)^A I_0$$

Where:

I is the radiation intensity after passing through a material that has thickness expressed in half-value layers

I_0 is the initial intensity of radiation

A is the number of half-value layers, which can be calculated by determining the thickness of the material and then dividing that number by material half-value layer

Use:

To characterize the attenuation ability (properties) of a material for shielding design or estimating exposures.

Example:

A source has a ¼ inch thick lead shield. The exposure rate at 1 foot from the unshielded source is 10 mR/hr. According to literature, the half-value layer is 0.25 cm. What is the exposure rate at 1 foot from the boxed source?

Step 1: Convert the shield to cm

$$.25 \text{ inch thick shield x } \frac{2.54\ cm}{inch} = 0.635 \text{ cm}$$

Step 2: Determine the number of half-value layers

$$Half\ value\ layers = \frac{0.635\ cm}{0.25\ cm}$$

$$Half\ value\ layers = 2.54$$

Solve for intensity (I)

$$I = \left(\frac{1}{2}\right)^A I_0$$

$$I = \left(\frac{1}{2}\right)^{2.54} 10mR/hr$$

$$I = 1.7 \text{ mR/hr}$$

Alternate Shield Thickness based on Half-Value Layer

$$X = 3.32 \, log \left(\frac{I_1}{I_2}\right) (HVL)$$

Where:

X is the necessary shield thickness

I_1 is the intensity of the initial radiation

I_2 is the intensity of the residual radiation

HVL is the thickness of the half-value layer

NOTE: The units for I_1 and I_2 must be the same and the units for x and HVL will be the same.

Use:

To design shield thickness to reduce intensity to a desired level or determine thickness based on the reduction of measured intensity.

Example:

The reactor maintenance group must build a lead wall to reduce worker exposure from 10 mR/hr to 0.25 mR/hr. Literature indicates the half-value layer is 0.5 cm. How thick must the lead wall be constructed to reach the desired level of reduction?

Step 1: Solve for X

$$X = 3.32 \, log \left(\frac{I_1}{I_2}\right) (HVL)$$

$$X = 3.32 \, log \left(\frac{10 \, mR/hr}{0.25 \, mR/hr}\right) (0.5 \, cm)$$

$$X = 2.65 \text{ cm}$$

Attenuation Half-Value

$$I_2 = \frac{I_1}{2^{\frac{x}{HLV}}}$$

Where:

I_2 is the intensity of the residual radiation after it has passed through a material that has a thickness expressed in half-value layers

I_1 is the initial intensity of the radiation

x is the thickness of the material

HVL is the thickness of the half-value layer

NOTE: The intensities must be expressed in consistent units and the thickness and half-value thickness must be in consistent units.

Use:

To design shield thickness to reduce intensity to a desired level, or determine thickness based on the reduction of measured intensity.

Example:

A radioisotope measured at one foot has an exposure rate of 15 millirem/hour. The isotope is stored in a 6 inch x 6 inch x 6 inch metal lock box. The box walls are ¼ inch thick. The half value layer is 0.4 cm for this condition. Calculate the exposure rate at one foot from the source when it is stored in the box.

Step 1: Convert the thickness of the wall to centimeters

$$.25 \text{ inches} \times \frac{2.54\ cm}{1\ inch}$$

$$= 0.635 \text{ cm}$$

Step 2: Solve for I_2

$$I_2 = \frac{I_1}{2^{\frac{x}{HLV}}}$$

$$I_2 = \frac{15\ millirem/hr}{2^{\frac{0.635\ cm}{0.4\ cm}}}$$

$$= 5 \text{ millirem/hr}$$

$$I = \left(\frac{1}{10}\right)^B I_0$$

Where:

I is the residual radiation intensity after it has passed through a material that has thickness expressed in tenth-value layers

I_0 is the initial intensity of the radiation

B is the thickness expressed as tenth-value layers (unitless)

Use:

An alternative to half-value for characterizing the attenuation ability (properties) of a material for shielding design or estimating exposures.

Example:

A radioisotope measured at one foot has an exposure rate of 15 millirem/hour. The isotope is stored in a 6 inch x 6 inch x 6 inch metal lock box. The box walls are ¼ inch thick. The tenth value layer is 0.85 cm for this condition. Calculate the exposure rate at one foot from the source when it is stored in the box.

Step 1: Convert the thickness of the wall to centimeters

$$.25 \text{ inches x } \frac{2.54\ cm}{1\ inch}$$

$$= 0.635 \text{ cm}$$

Step 2: Solve for the number of tenth-value layers, B

$$B = \frac{0.635\ cm}{0.85\ cm}$$

$$B = 0.747$$

Step 3: Solve for I

$$I = \left(\frac{1}{10}\right)^B I_0$$

$$I = \left(\frac{1}{10}\right)^{0.747} 15\ millirem/hr$$

$$I = 2.69\ millirem/hour$$

$$I_2 = \frac{I_1}{10^{\frac{x}{TVL}}}$$

Where:

I_2 is the residual radiation intensity after it has passed through a material

I_1 is the initial radiation intensity radiation

x is the thickness of the material

TVL is the thickness of the tenth-value layer (same units as x)

Use:

An alternative to half-value for characterizing the attenuation ability (properties) of a material.

Example:

A source is stored in a metal cabinet 2 cm thick. The exposure rate at 1 foot from the unshielded source is 10 mR/hr. According to literature, the tenth-value layer is 0.05 cm. What is the exposure rate at 1 foot from the boxed source?

Step 1: Solve for I_2

$$I_2 = \frac{I_1}{10^{\frac{x}{TVL}}}$$

$$I_2 = \frac{10mR/hr}{10^{\frac{2\ cm}{0.05\ cm}}}$$

$$I_2 = 1 \times 10^{-39} \text{ mR/hr}$$

$$D = \frac{\Gamma A}{d^2}$$

Where:

D is the rate of exposure

Γ is the gamma ray constant $\frac{R-cm^2}{mCi-hr}$ and is dependent on the radionuclide used as the gamma source

A is the activity of the source, typically expressed as (mCi)

d is the distance from the source, expressed as (cm)

Use:

To calculate exposure rate at different distances from known activities.

Example:

Calculate the exposure rate at 2 feet from a 10 mCi source of Iodine 131, that has gamma constant of 2.2 R/mCi-hr at 1 cm.

Step 1: Convert the distance to centimeters

$$2\ feet \ x \ \frac{2.54\ cm}{inch} \ x \ \frac{12\ inches}{foot}$$

$$= 60.96\ cm$$

Step 2: Solve for the exposure rate, D

$$D = \frac{\Gamma A}{d^2}$$

$$D = 2.2 \frac{R - cm^2}{mCi - hr} \frac{10\ mCi}{(60.96cm)^2}$$

D = 0.0059 rem/hr or 5.9 mrem/hr

Exponential Attenuation

$$I = I_0 B e^{-\mu x}$$

Where:
I is the intensity of attenuated radiation
I₀ is the initial intensity of radiation on a material
B is the unitless build-up factor that is dependent on the material
e is the log base e
μ is the attenuation coefficient, expressed as (cm⁻¹)
x is the thickness of the material, expressed as (cm)
Use:
Determining the penetration of radiation through a material while accounting for scattered radiation by using the build-up factor.

Example:
The measured gamma radiation exposure rate for a source is 3 millirem/hour. The radiation control department has provided an iron box with 2-inch thick walls for storing the source. The gamma radiation energy for the source is 0.6 MeV. The attenuation coefficient and build up factor for iron is obtained from the literature: 0.5 cm⁻¹ and 4.0 for 2 inches. Calculate the remaining radiation intensity.

Step 1: Step 1: Convert the thickness to centimeters

$$2\ inches \times \frac{2.54\ cm}{inch}$$

$$= 5.08\ cm$$

Step 2: Solve for e⁻ᵘˣ

$$e^{-0.47\,(5.08)} = 0.092$$

Step 3: Solve for the intensity of the attenuated radiation, I

$$I = I_0 B e^{-\mu x}$$

$$I = 3\ millirem(4.0)(092)$$

$$I = 1.1\ millirem/hour$$

$$\frac{1}{T_{1/2eff}} = \frac{1}{T_{1/2rad}} + \frac{1}{T_{1/2bio}}$$

Where:

$T_{1/2eff}$ is the effective half-life of radioactive material in an organism

$T_{1/2rad}$ is the radiological half-life of a source

T_{bio} is the biological half-life for a material based on time of metabolism and excretion

NOTE: The units must be consistent between the half-lives.

Use:

To calculate the rate at which radioactivity decreases in the body, which allows for calculation of the dose.

Rearranged->

$$T_{1/2eff} = \frac{(T_{1/2rad})(T_{1/2bio})}{T_{1/2rad} + T_{1/2bio}}$$

Example:

What is the effective half-life for polonium-210 internal exposure? The radiological half-life is 138 days, and according to literature, the biological half-life is approximately 40 days.

Step 1: Use the rearranged formula and solve for $T_{1/2eff}$

$$T_{1/2eff} = \frac{(T_{1/2rad})(T_{1/2bio})}{T_{1/2rad} + T_{1/2bio}}$$

$$T_{1/2eff} = \frac{(138 \ days)(40 \ days)}{138 \ days + 40 \ days}$$

$$T_{1/2eff} = 31 \ days$$

Note: As the biological half-life increases, the exposure to the isotope increases.

Rubric 13: Ionizing Radiation Questions

1. Gamma rays originate in the nucleus and travel at the speed of light. This highly penetrating radiation interacts with matter in three ways. Select the answer that <u>does not</u> describe a method of interaction for gamma rays.

    A) Photoelectric effect
    B) Pair production
    C) Scintillation
    D) Compton effect

2. A source is producing 125 mR/hour at 1 meter. Workers must perform repairs in the same room as the source but must not be exposed to more than 1 mR for the hour that the repair task will require. What distance must be maintained from the source by the workers to prevent the exposure from being unacceptable during the task?

    A) 11.2 m
    B) 0.9 m
    C) 110 m
    D) 11 m

3. The splitting of an atomic nucleus, and the release of energy and radioactive materials is called:

    A) Explosion
    B) Fission
    C) Fusion
    D) Disintegration

4. The field of radiobiology began when two French biologists began studying the effect of radiation on frog eggs. The work of the biologists has been generalized as the "Law of Bergonie and Tribondeau." The basic conclusion of their study is:

    A) The intensity of the radiation decreases with the square of the distance.
    B) The rapid slowing of beta radiation results in a secondary release of gamma radiation.
    C) The dose of the radiation is proportional to the intensity of the radiation.
    D) The sensitivity of a tissue is proportional to the reproductive activity.

5. A worker is exposed to a radium source, which is an alpha emitter, with an estimated absorbed dose of 0.15 mrad/hour. Calculate the estimated dose equivalent for a 7-hour exposure.

Source	Quality Factor
X-ray	1.0
Gamma	1.0
Beta	1.0
Alpha	20
Slow neutron	10
Fast neutron	30

A) 0.021 rem
B) 0.02 mrem
C) 3.0 mrem
D) 0.003 rad

6. In 1949, the ICRP introduced the 'standard man' concept. What was the purpose of the 'standard man?'

A) Ergonomic design reference.
B) To standardize the mass of important human organs and tissues.
C) To standardize facial sizes for respiratory protection.
D) To reference the development of threshold limit values for the ACGIH.

7. Select the best description of the Linear, No Threshold hypothesis.

A) A mathematical relationship between the severity of the radiation effect and the total dose.
B) The value of response is related to the median exposure effect.
C) Low energy transfer is linear and does not produce a radiation effect threshold.
D) Control of radiation doses for the purpose of limiting potential effects.

8. There are several factors related to radiation exposure and biological damage. Select the factors that result in the greatest biological effect.

A) Increase the dose, exposure to the arms, hands, and fingers.
B) Expose to a larger surface area.
C) Increase the area of exposure, exposure includes internal organs.
D) Increase the dose, decrease the area of exposure.

9. Radon is a noble gas linked to cancer in humans when exposed to high doses. Select the cancer related to radon exposure.

   A) Brain
   B) Leukemia
   C) Ovarian
   D) Lung

10. A popular personal radiation-monitoring device utilizes small salt chips. This detector is a _____.

    A) Thermoluminescent detector
    B) Film badge
    C) Silver iodide film detector
    D) Scintillation chamber

11. The gamma radiation at 20 cm from an I-125 source is measured at 100 millirem/hour. The lead half-value layer is 0.0043 cm. What thickness of lead placed 20 cm from the source will lower the gamma radiation to 2 millirem/hour?

    A) 0.015 cm
    B) 0.024 cm
    C) 0.180 cm
    D) 0.400 cm

12. What is the absorbed dose of high-energy protons if the absorbed dose in rad is equal to 1 rem?

    A) 0.1
    B) 1
    C) 5
    D) 10

13. Intact skin provides a shield to which type of ionizing radiation?

    A) Alpha
    B) Beta
    C) Gamma
    D) X-rays

14. Which of the following cell types is least susceptible to radiosensitivity?

    A) Lymphocytes
    B) Nerve cells
    C) Gastric gland cells
    D) Osteoblast cells

15. What is the function of an annular impactor head?

    A) Trap airborne particles.
    B) Collect airborne contamination.
    C) Collect surface contamination.
    D) Absorb liquid particles that are filterable.

16. The half-life of iodine-131 is 8.02 days. The biological half-life of iodine in the thyroid is approximately 115 days. The activity level of iodine in a person's thyroid on March 1 is 35 microcuries. What is the estimated activity level in the person's thyroid on April 1?

    A) 0.45 microcuries
    B) 1.99 microcuries
    C) 5.59 microcuries
    D) 10.34 microcuries

17. What is the key method(s) for protection against external sources of radiation?

    A) Keep at maximum distance from the radiation source.
    B) Stay near the radiation source only for the shortest possible time.
    C) Shield the radiation source.
    D) All of the above.

18. There are three types of gas-filled detectors. Each detector contains a central wire known as a(n) _____ , which initially carries a _____ charge.

    A) Anode; positive.
    B) Lace; positive.
    C) Anode; negative.
    D) Lace; negative.

19. Cesium-137 is a radioactive isotope material with a half-life of 30.17 years, and the gamma ray constant is 2.60 R-cm2/mCi-hr. The activity of the source is 3 microcuries. Estimate the radiation dose from the cesium-137 during a 3-hour exposure at a distance of approximately 20 feet from the source.

    A) 0.029 microREM
    B) 0.063 microREM
    C) 12.9 microREM
    D) 36.1 milliREM

20. In regard to the shielding equation shown below, what if μ is larger than the shielding material for the photon energy of interest?

$$I = I_0 B e^{-\mu x}$$

    A. A material shall have undermined shielding properties.
    B. No more effective than if μ were smaller.
    C. A more effective shield.
    D. A less effective shield.

Rubric 13: Ionizing Radiation Answers

1. Answer: C
Explanation: Scintillation is a class of radiation detection based on the energy transmission from radiation to a substance that responds to this energy transfer by emitting light. Photoelectric effect is the process of a gamma photon ejecting an electron and transferring most of the energy to the electron. The Compton Effect is the process of a gamma photon ejecting an electron and a reduced energy photon, which may cause additional ionization. In pair production, the gamma photon enters the vicinity of a nucleus without striking it, causing an electron and positron to be created. *Source: Industrial Hygiene Reference and Study Guide, 3rd edition*

2. Answer: A
Explanation: The task will take 1 hour, so the unit of time for the exposure is equivalent.

Step 1: Use the inverse square law to solve for the distance

$$\frac{I_1}{I_2} = \left[\frac{d_2}{d_1}\right]^2$$

$$\frac{1.25 \; mr/Hr}{1 \; mR/Hr} = \left[\frac{d_2}{1 \; meter}\right]^2$$

$$\sqrt{1.25x1 \; m^2} = d_2$$

$$11.2 \; m = d_2$$

Rounding down to 11 would allow the dose to exceed 1 mR per hour; therefore, use 11.2 or round up to 12 if 11.2 is not a choice.

3. Answer: B
Explanation: This is a definition of fission, which typically occurs with uranium-233, uranium-235 and plutonium-239.

4. Answer: D
Explanation: The "Law of Bergonie and Tribondeau" states the radiosensitivity of a tissue is directly proportional to the reproductive activity and inversely proportional to the degree of differentiation, which applies to most mammalian cells. *Source: The Occupational Environment: Its Evaluation, Control and Management, 3rd Edition*

5. Answer: A
Explanation:

Source	Quality Factor
X-ray	1.0
Gamma	1.0
Beta	1.0
Alpha	20
Slow neutron	10
Fast neutron	30

Step 1: Locate the QF factor for Alpha particles: 20

Step 2: Solve for REM

$$rem = rad \times QF$$

$$rem = 0.15 \text{ mrad/hour} \times 20 \text{ mrem/mrad} \times 7 \text{ hours}$$

$$= 21 \text{ mrem or } 0.021 \text{ rem}$$

Source: Useful Equations: Practical Applications of OH & S Math, 3rd Edition

6. Answer: B
Explanation: The standard man model specifies the mass of organs and tissues for use with radiation dose and response determination. It was revised in 1959 to include distribution of the elements in the total body and effective radii of all the organs, including intake and excretion rates. The model is now referred to as the 'reference man.' The reference man is 70 kg, 1.7 m tall, 20-30 years old, Caucasian male, in temperate climate with US – Northern European habits. *Source: The Occupational Environment: Its Evaluation, Control and Management, 3rd Edition*

7. Answer: D
Explanation: The hypothesis states that scientists have observed a linear relationship between radiation dose and effect at high doses, and it is assumed that for radiation protection purposes, the relationship for low doses is also linear. This hypothesis has been adopted by all national and international radiation protection organizations. *Source: The Occupational Environment: Its Evaluation, Control and Management, 3rd Edition*

8. Answer: C
Explanation: The biological effects are related to the exposure. More exposure (dose) increases the effect. The area of the body exposed is important: The extremities are less sensitive to radiation than the torso because no critical organs are in the extremities. Rapidly dividing cells are the most sensitive. Accordingly, the embryo or fetus is considered most sensitive. Likewise, children are more sensitive than adults. *Source: The Occupational Environment: Its Evaluation, Control and Management, 3rd Edition*

9. Answer: D
Explanation: The EPA estimates 5,000-20,000 cases of lung cancer per year are related to inhalation of radon. If radon decays while inhaled, progeny are produced, all of which emit high-energy alpha radiation that causes lung damage.

10. Answer: A
Explanation: TLDs may have several salt chips or elements for different dose monitoring requirements. They are small, light, and easy to handle. They can detect a broad range of exposures. TLDs can only be read once.

11. Answer: B

$$X = 3.32 \, log\left(\frac{I_1}{I_2}\right)(HVL)$$

X is the shield thickness
I_1 is the incident intensity
I_2 is the exit intensity
HVL is the half-value layer

Step 1: Solve for X

$$X = 3.32 log\left(\frac{100 \, millirem/hour}{2 \, millirem/hour}\right)(0.0043 \, cm)$$

$$X = 0.024 \, cm$$

Source: None provided

12. Answer: A
Explanation:

Table: Quality Factors and Absorbed Dose Equivalencies		
Type of Radiation	**Quality factor (Q)**	**Absorbed dose equal to a unit**
X-, gamma, or beta radiation	1	1
Alpha particles	20	0.05
Neutrons of unknown energy	10	0.1
High-energy protons	10	0.1
Note: Absorbed dose in rad equal to 1 rem or the absorbed dose in gray equal to 1 sievert		

Source: nrc.gov

13. Answer: A
Explanation: Alpha particles are charged particles that are emitted from naturally occurring materials and man-made elements. Alpha particles have a very limited ability to penetrate other materials. These particles of ionizing radiation can be blocked by a sheet of paper, skin, or even a few inches of air. Alpha-radiation is completely stopped by the skin and thus does not injure skin. *Source: nrc.gov and Fundamentals of Industrial Hygiene*

14. Answer: B
Explanation: The damage to cells depends on three factors. These factors include reproductive activity, mitotic activity, and differentiation. Types of cells in order of susceptibility (most susceptible to least susceptible) are listed as follows: Lymphocytes; Granulosa cells; Myelocytes; Gastric gland cells; Endothelial; Osteoblasts; Chondroblasts; Granulocytes; Osteocytes; Erythrocytes; Fibrocytes; Phagocytes; Muscle cells; and Nerve cells. *Source: Radiation Protection: A Practical Guide, Engelhardt & Associates*

15. Answer: A
Explanation: An annular impactor head collects alpha, beta, and gamma emitting contaminants. An annular kinetic impactor head collects large airborne particles. The device does not collect radon and thoron. The approximate efficiency is 95%. *Source: energy.gov*

16. Answer: B
Explanation:
Step 1: Determine the effective half-life of iodine-131 in the thyroid

$$T_{\frac{1}{2}eff} = \frac{\left(T_{\frac{1}{2}rad}\right)\left(T_{\frac{1}{2}bio}\right)}{T_{\frac{1}{2}rad} + T_{\frac{1}{2}bio}}$$

$$T_{\frac{1}{2}eff} = \frac{(8.02\ days)(115\ days)}{8.02\ days + 115\ days}$$

$$T_{\frac{1}{2}eff} = 7.50\ days$$

Step 2: Determine the activity level after 31 days

$$A = A_i(0.5)^{\frac{t}{T_{\frac{1}{2}}}}$$

$$A = 35\ \mu Ci(0.5)^{\frac{31}{7.50}}$$

$$A = 1.99\ \mu Ci$$

17. **Answer: D**

Explanation: There are several ways to protect oneself from external sources of radiation. The three most important are concepts of time, distance, and shielding. Keep at a maximum distance from the source (distance); avoid radiation sources when possible, and limit the amount of time spent around a radiation source (time); and shield the radiation source when possible. *Source: The Occupational Environment: Its Evaluation, Control and Management, 3rd edition*

18. **Answer: A**

Explanation: There are three types of gas-filled detectors: Geiger counters or Geiger Mueller detectors; Proportional counters; and Ionization Chambers. Each contains a central wire known as an anode, which initially carries a positive (+) charge. Alpha and beta particle interactions inside the gas produce primarily ion pairs. The electron component of the ion pair will be attracted to the anode. The positive member of the ion pair will be attracted to the outer wall, which is initially negatively (-) charged with respect to the anode (e.g., cathode). Gamma ray interactions will occur first within the cathode wall rather than the fill gas. These interactions will eject electrons from the wall that then ionize the gas. *Source: The Occupational Environment: Its Evaluation, Control, and Management, 3rd Edition*

19. **Answer: B**

Explanation: The gamma-ray constant equation can be used to estimate exposure.

$$D = \frac{\Gamma A}{d^2}$$

Step 1: Solve for D

$$D = \frac{\left(2.60 \frac{R-cm^2}{mCi-hr}\right)(0.003\ mCi)}{\left(20\ feet\left(\frac{30.48\ cm}{ft}\right)\right)^2}$$

$$D = 21.0 x 10^{-9} \frac{R}{hr}$$

$$D = 21.0 x\ 10^{-3} \frac{\mu rem}{hr}$$

Step 2: Solve for Total Dose

$$Total\ dose = dose\ rate\ x\ time$$

$$Total\ dose = 21.0\ x\ 10^{-3} \frac{\mu rem}{hr}\ x\ 3\ hours$$

$$Total\ dose = 0.063\ \mu rem$$

20. Answer: C

$$I = I_0 B e^{-\mu x}$$

Explanation: This equation calculates the attenuation when a shield is placed between a detector and a point source of x or γ rays. The linear attenuation coefficient (μ) is strongly dependent on the shield composition and energy of the radiation. The shield becomes more effective as the interacting portion grows larger. *Source: Useful Equations for Radiation, Wright State University*

Rubric 14: Non-ionizing Radiation

Non-ionizing radiation includes ultraviolet (UV), visible, infrared (IR), radio frequency and extremely low frequency (ELF) fields. Typically, non-ionizing radiation is defined as having less than 12 electron volts (eV) energy, which is the level at which the energy can cause ionization of atoms. Accordingly, ionizing radiation is defined as having 12 eV or more energy.

Radiation and Wavelength

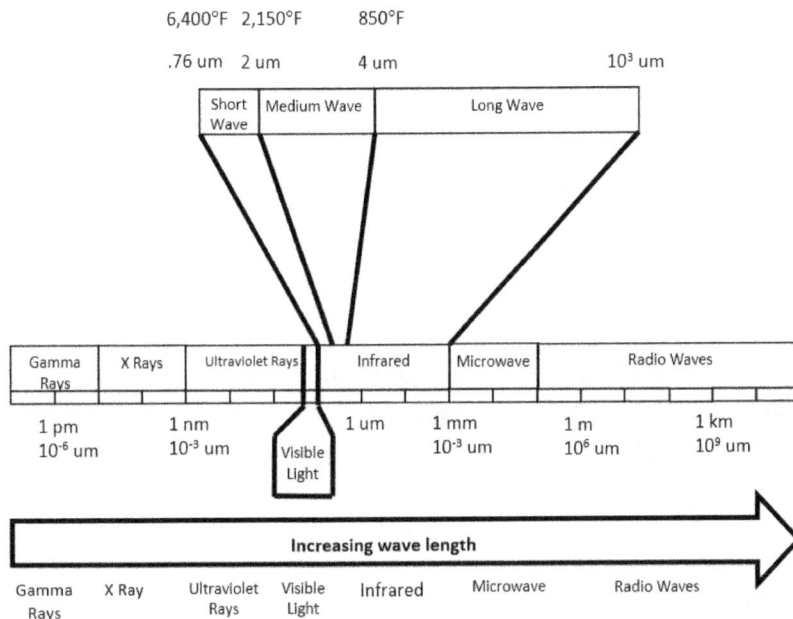

Span Image

Important Terms and Definitions

Absolute Gain (G) - Gain (g) is a measure of the directional properties of an antenna that represents the increase in power output of a system in relation to an ideal isotropic emitter. For a point source antenna, the gain is 1, but if a reflector is added, the radiation pattern is changed and the gain is greater than 1. When gain is used in calculations, values of **absolute gain (G)** must be used: $G = 10^{g/10}$.

Aphakic – Without a lens. Workers who have had the lens of their eye removed are at a greater risk of retinal photochemical injury.

Conjunctivitis – Inflammation of the membrane that lines the eyelids and covers the exposed surface of the eyeball.

Erythema- Reddening of the skin.

Frequency – The rate at which oscillations are produced. Expressed as Hertz (Hz), which is equivalent to one cycle per second.

Lambertian reflectance is the property that defines an ideal "matte" or diffusely reflecting surface. The apparent brightness of a **Lambertian surface** to an observer is the same regardless of the observer's angle of view.

Melanoma - A type of cancer that develops from the pigment-containing cells known as melanocytes. It is primarily related to UV exposure.

Nominal Hazard Zone (NHZ) – A zone based on distance that defines the distance from the source of laser exposure to a distance at which eye exposure is considered safe.

Optical Density (OD) – The quantity used to specify the ability of protective eyewear to attenuate optical radiation.

Phosphenes – Visual sensations of flickering white light.

Photokeratitis – An injury to the eye that results from acute, high-intensity exposure to UV-B and UV-C.

Photon Energy (eV or ergs) - An elementary particle, the quantum of all forms of electromagnetic radiation, including light. It is the force carrier for electromagnetic force. It is expressed as E = Plank's constant x frequency.

Photosensitization – Reaction to light that includes phototoxicity and photoallergy.

Planck's Constant – 4.13×10^{-15} eV-sec

Power Density (PD) – The measure of radiant power per area, typically mW/cm^2. Also known as irradiance and is the cross product of E and H field vectors. Increasing field strength will increase the PD, but will not increase the photon energy

Radiance – The radiometric brightness of an extended source.

Wavelength – The measured distance between two analogous points on two successive points of a wave (i.e. peak to peak).

Non-Ionizing Radiation

Non-Ionizing Radiation: Wavelength or Frequency

REGION	WAVELENGTH	FREQUENCY
Ultraviolet	100 – 400 nm	-
• UV-C	• 100 – 280 nm	-
• UV-B	• 280 – 320 nm	-
• UV-A	• 320 – 400 nm	-
Visible	400 – 770 nm	-
Infrared	770 nm – 1000 um (1 mm)	-
• IR-A	• 770 – 1400 nm (1.4 um)	-
• IR-B	• 1.4 um – 3 um	-
• IR-C	• 3 um – 15 um	-
○ Far IR	• 15 um – 1000 um (1 mm)	-
Radio Frequency	-	300 GHz – 3 KHz
Extremely Low Frequency	-	3KHz – 3 Hz

Example:
Which of the non-ionizing radiation groups is described by wavelength?
- a) UV-A, UV-B, ELF
- b) UV, Radio
- c) UV, Visible, ELF
- d) UV, IR

Answer: D.
Explanation: UV, IR and Laser radiation are described by wavelength, while radio frequency and extremely low frequency are described by frequency. Although not as great a health hazard as ionizing radiation, non-ionizing radiation does have biological effects related to exposure.

Biological Effects of Non-Ionizing Radiation

SPECTRAL REGION	TARGET ORGAN	MAJOR EFFECT
ELF	• Eyes • Skin • Nervous system	• Behavioral changes • Phosphenes • Shock, burns
RF	• Nervous system • Reproductive system • Eyes • Skin	• Behavioral changes • Malformations • Cataracts • Burns
IR	• Eyes • Skin	• Retinal lesions, cataracts • Burns
VISIBLE	• Eyes • Skin	• Retinal lesions • Burns
UV	• Immune system • Eyes • Skin	• Photokeratitis • Conjunctivitis • Cataracts

Ultraviolet

The predominant source of UV exposure is sunlight. UV exposure can be related to xenon lights, welding and tanning bed usage. Ultraviolet has the highest photon energy range but penetration is limited. Target organs are the skin and cornea. The health effects are delayed, with no immediate sensation of injury. UVA (near UV) are the UV frequencies near the visible frequencies. UVB (actinic UV) are mid frequencies and considered the most damaging. UVC (far UV) is also known as vacuum UV. UV is measured with a photosensitive cell with appropriate filters (UV meter).

Visible

Visible light is necessary for the process of vision. Sources include sunlight and generated sources, including light bulbs, welding, lasers and other illumination devices. Target organs are skin and eye. Ocular pain is associated with exposure to blue light (0.425 – 0.450 nm wavelength). Visible light is measured with a photosensitive cell (light meter).

Infrared

Sources of IR radiation include welding, metal and other industrial furnaces, sunlight and arc lamps. The health effects are primary effects, including localized skin burn and conjunctivitis. Glass Blower's cataracts. IR-A penetrates the skin, and the eye to the retina. IR-B is mostly absorbed by outer layers of skin and eye. IR-C causes skin burns, corneal burns and cataract formation, and is measured with a photosensitive cell.

Radio Frequency & Microwave Radiation

Radio frequencies are used in navigation; radio; heat sealers and radar; and for scientific and medical purposes. The health effects are primarily associated with thermal effects, such as whole body or localized heating, but some immune system and endocrine (Pearl Chain formation) effects can occur.

This type of energy is measured with a dipole antenna for electric field and loop antenna for magnetic field.

Microwave sources include cooking with ovens, televisions, and radar. The health effects include thermal heating. Shorter wavelengths increase surface temperature and longer wavelengths penetrate deeper. Microwave exposure is associated with cataract formation. It is measured with calibrated dipole antenna that measures electric field strength.

Extremely Low Frequency

Low frequency radiation is associated with generating, transmitting and using electricity, as well as induction furnaces. Exposure limits for extremely low electric fields, magnetic fields and contact currents are typically voluntary guidelines or standards due to the lack of definitive dose-response evidence and epidemiological studies that support biological effects in humans.

Current exposure recommendations are based on effects to the central nervous system. Very little energy is absorbed at the common US Power frequency of 60 HZ. There is a possible, but not-conclusive, link to childhood leukemia. Electric fields (E fields) are measured with a free-body dipole probe.

Lasers

LASER is an acronym for *Light Amplification by Stimulated Emission of Radiation*. The radiation produced emerges from the LASER as a beam. The beam is powerful, monochromatic, directional and coherent.

Lasers are classified according to the potential hazard produced. In accordance with IEC 69825-1 Second Edition, the classes are listed below:

- *Class 1*
  - Laser products that are safe during use, including long-term direct intrabeam viewing, even while using optical viewing instruments. It also includes fully enclosed high-power lasers.
- *Class 1M*
  - Laser products that are safe for long-term direct intrabeam viewing for the naked eye. Eye injury may occur if optical viewing instruments are used with 100 mm for diverging beams and certain collimated beams.
- *Class 2*
  - Laser products that emit visible light radiation in the wavelength range of 400 nm to 700 nm that are safe for momentary exposures but can be hazardous for deliberate beam viewing.
- *Class 2M*
  - Laser products that emit visible beams and are safe for short time exposure only for the naked eye. Eye injury may occur if optical viewing instruments are used with 100 mm for diverging beams and certain collimated beams.

- *Class 3R*
  - Laser products that emit radiation that can exceed maximum permissible exposures during direct intrabeam viewing, but the risk is low because of the required exposure durations.

- *Class 3B*
  - Laser products that are normally hazardous when intrabeam ocular exposure occurs within the Nominal Ocular Hazard Distance (NOHD), including accidental short duration exposures. Specular reflections of these beams may be hazardous, although diffuse reflections are usually considered safe. May produce skin injuries or ignite flammable materials.

- *Class 4*
  - Laser products that are hazardous when intrabeam and diffuse reflections are viewed. Skin exposure is hazardous. Often ignites flammable materials.

Laser Induced Eye Damage

LASER SPECTRAL REGION	TARGET STRUCTURE	RELATIVE PENETRATION
IR-A	Retina, Lens	Moderate to Maximum
IR-B	Cornea, Lens	Shallow
IR-C	Cornea	Topical
VISIBLE	Retina	Maximum
UV- C	Cornea	Topical
UV-B	Lens, Cornea	Shallow
UV-A	Retina, Lens	Moderate

Exposure guidelines have been published by ANSI, ACGIH, ICNIRP, and IEC. These guidelines express limits for skin and eye exposure and are wavelength dependent.

Field measurements of laser radiation is not recommended due to difficulty in obtaining meaningful measurements. Rather than measure, the hazards are evaluated by using a numerical method. The Maximum Permissible Exposure Limit (MPE) is defined in ANSI Z136.1. The MPE is then used to calculate the Nominal Hazard Zone (NHZ), the primary hazard evaluation method when there is access to an open beam.

Non-Ionizing Radiation Equations

Frequency – Wavelength Relationship

$$f = \frac{c}{\lambda}$$

Where:

f is the frequency, expressed as (Hz)

c is the speed of light, expressed as (m/sec or cm/sec)

λ lambda is the wavelength (m or cm).

Note: Speed of light 3.0 x 10^8 m/sec or 9.8 x 10^8 f/sec.

Use:

Determining either frequency or wavelength when one of two is known.

Example:

A field is determined to be at 60 Hz. What is the wavelength?

$$f = \frac{c}{\lambda}$$

$$f = \frac{9.8 \; x \; 10^8 \; ft/sec}{60 \; c/sec}$$

$$f = 1.6 \; x \; 10^8 \; c/sec$$

Photon Energy

$$E = f \; x \; h$$

Where:

E is the photon energy, expressed as ergs or eV-sec

f is frequency, expressed as (cycles/sec or Hz)

h is Planck's constant energy (6.626 x 10^{-27} erg-sec or 4.13 x 10^{-15} eV-sec).

Use:

To calculate photon energy

Example:

What is the photon energy for a 120Hz source?

$$E = f \; x \; h$$

$$E = 120 \; x \; 4.13 \; x \; 10^{-15} \; \text{eV-sec}$$

$$E = 4.96 \; x \; 10^{-13} \; \text{eV-sec}$$

Optical Density – Eye Protection Selection

$$O.D = \log\left[\frac{ML}{EL}\right]$$

Where:

O.D. is the optical density used to specify the ability of the eye protection (unitless)

ML is the measured or calculated level of irradiance or optical radiation

EL is the exposure limit for optical radiation

Use: Calculating the protection level required for the eyewear to be effective at attenuating the optical radiation.

Note: Both ML and EL are measures of irradiance or optical radiation and the calculation must have similar terms, typically mW/cm^2.

Example:

Optical density levels range from 1 to 8 with corresponding attenuation levels of 10 to 100,000,000. If the measured irradiance level is 120 mW/cm^2, and the exposure limit is 0.0190 mW/cm^2, what is the minimal level of optical density required for the protective eyewear?

$$O.D = \log\left[\frac{ML}{EL}\right]$$

$$O.D. = \log\left[\frac{120 mW/cm^2}{0.190\ mW/cm^2}\right]$$

$$O.D. = 2.8$$

Note: If selecting eyewear based on whole number O.D. values, round up to 3.

Optical Density - Field Test

$$O.D. = \log\left[\frac{I_0}{I}\right]$$

Where:

O.D. is the calculated optical density

I_0 is the measured optical irradiance at the eye **without** eye protection

I is the measured optical irradiance at the eye **with** eye protection

Use: Calculating the effective attenuation of the eye protection

UV Effective Irradiance

$$t = \frac{0.003 \, J/cm^2}{E_{eff}}$$

Where:
t is the allowed time of exposure (seconds).
J is one Joule (1 watt-sec).
E_{eff} is the effective irradiance (W/cm^2) relative to a monochromatic source at 270 nm.
Use: Calculate the allowed exposure time to UV radiation.

Example:
The safety and health technician uses a photometer and determines that the potential effective irradiance exposure is 60 uW/cm^2. What is the allowed duration of unprotected eye and skin exposure during an 8-hour work shift? (*Note*: This applies to UV across the 200-315 nm wavelength range; a separate measurement would be made for longer wavelengths.)

$$t = \frac{0.003 \, J/cm^2}{E_{eff}}$$

Step 1: Convert 60 uW/cm^2 to W/cm^2

$$\frac{60 \, uW}{cm^2} \, x \, \frac{1 \, W}{1000000 uW} = 0.0006 \, \frac{W}{cm^2}$$

Step 2: Solve for allowable time t (seconds)

$$t = \frac{0.003 \, J/cm^2}{0.0006 \dfrac{W}{cm^2}}$$

$$t = 50 \text{ seconds}$$

Magnetic Field Coils

Magnetic fields are commonly measured by magnetic field coils. The device sensitivity is related to the area or number of loops. Typically, the device is oriented in the field of interest to obtain a maximum reading. Alternatively, the magnitude of the flux density **B**, which is the amount of magnetic flux through a unit area taken perpendicular to the direction of the magnetic flux, can be calculated from three measurements taken at right angles to each other as shown below.

Magnetic Field Flux Density

$$B = \sqrt{B_x^2 + B_y^2 + B_z^2}$$

Where:
B is the magnetic field flux density, expressed as (tesla)
$B_{x,y,z}$ are the measured flux densities obtained from three different planes, expressed as (tesla)
Use: Calculating flux density based on coiled loop survey measurements for comparison to recommended limits. Applies to the magnetic element of ELF.
Note: The measurement technique has been improved with modern orthogonal coils and electronic circuitry.

Example:
The 2015 ACGIH TLV book lists the whole-body TLV for magnetic flux density in the 1 to 300 Hz range as $B_{tlv}= 60/f$. This is a ceiling limit expressed as millitesla (mT). The technician records the flux densities from three different planes as: $B_x= 0.3$ mT, $B_y = 0.5$ mT, $B_z = 2$ mT. What is the magnetic flux density for the 60Hz source and is the TLV exceeded?

Step 1: Calculate the magnetic field density

$$B = \sqrt{B_x^2 + B_y^2 + B_z^2}$$

$$B = \sqrt{0.3_x^2 + 0.5_y^2 + 2_z^2}$$

$$B = 2mT$$

Step 2: Calculate the TLV

$$B_{tlv}= 60/f$$

$$B_{tlv}= 60/60$$

$$B_{tlv}= 1mT$$

The measured level of 2mT exceeds the TLV of 1 mT

Spatial Averaging of Either Electric or Magnetic Field Strength

$$spatial\ average = \left(\frac{\sum_{i=1}^{N} FS_i^2}{N}\right)^{\frac{1}{2}}$$

Where:

N is the number of measurements to be averaged. Ten (10) is the minimum recommended.

FS_i is either the electric or magnetic field strengths at i locations, (V/m or A/m).

Use: Allows for averaging of field measurements obtained in the 'operator absent' condition, which can then be used to estimate whole body exposure.

Example:

Ten electronic field measurements are taken at a location (operator absent). The results are shown below. Calculate the spatial average.

Step 1: Calculate the E-field^2 values

Location	E-field (V/m)	E-field^2 (V/m)^2
1	4	16
2	8	64
3	10	100
4	8	64
5	10	100
6	20	400
7	15	225
8	10	100
9	5	25
10	5	25
N = 10		Sum =1119

Step 2: Solve for the spatial average

$$spatial\ average = \left(\frac{\sum_{i=1}^{N} FS_i^2}{N}\right)^{\frac{1}{2}}$$

$$spatial\ average = \left(\frac{1119}{10}\right)^{1/2}$$

$$spatial\ average = 10.6\ V/m$$

Near Field Power Density

$$S = \frac{4P}{A}$$

Where:
S is the near field power density, expressed as (W/m^2 or mW/cm^2).
P is the power output from the antenna, expressed as (W).
A is the area of the antenna, expressed as (m^2).
Use: Calculate an estimate of near field power density.

Example:
Calculate the approximate near field power density for a dish antenna with a diameter of 2 meters and a radiated power of 200 W. The antenna is operating at a frequency of 1.3 GHz and λ of 23 cm.

Step 1: Calculate the area of the antenna.

$$A = \pi r^2$$

$$A = \pi 1^2$$

$$A = 3.1 m^2$$

Step 2: Solve for near field power density (W)

$$S = \frac{4P}{A}$$

$$S = \frac{4(200W)}{3.1 m^2}$$

$$S = 258 \ W/m^2$$

Power Density & Electric Field Strength

$$S = \frac{E^2}{3770}$$

Where:

S is the power density (mW/cm^2).

E is the electric field strength, i.e. the intensity of the electric field at a specific distance (V/m).

3770 is the far-field plane wave impedance value of 377Ω x 10.

Use: Allows for conversion of measured electrical field strength to power density, since power density is very difficult to measure directly.

Example:

The technician uses a calibrated stick antenna to measure the electric field. If the electric field is 150 V/m, calculate the power density.

$$S = \frac{E^2}{3770}$$

$$S = \frac{(150V/m)^2}{3770}$$

$$S = 5.97 \text{ mW/cm}^2$$

$$S = 37.7H^2$$

Where:

S is the power density, expressed as (mW/cm^2).

H is the magnetic field strength, expressed as amperes/meter (A/m).

37.7 is the far-field plane wave impedance value of 377Ω / 10.

Use: Allows for conversion of measured magnetic field strength to power density, since power density is difficult to measure directly.

Example:

The technician uses a calibrated loop antenna and measures the magnetic field. The magnetic field strength is 0.4 A/m. Calculate the power density.

$$S = 37.7H^2$$

$$S = 37.7(0.4A/m)^2$$

$$S = 6.0 \text{ mW/cm}^2$$

ANTENNA EQUATIONS

The following antenna equations may be associated with radio and microwave frequencies, such as radar, cellular, and microwave communications.

Absolute Gain – Antenna

$$G = 10^{g/10}$$

Where:

G is absolute gain, the ratio of transmitted power density to power density of a theoretical isotropic generator (dimensionless).

g is gain, a measure of the directional properties of an antenna, typically expressed as (dB).

Note: When gain is defined as decibels, absolute gain = G = $10^{(g/10)}$

Use: Calculation of safe distances from antennae.
Conversion of gain in dB to absolute value.

Example:

An antenna system has a measured gain of 35dB and an emitted power of 4500W. Calculate the absolute gain.

$$\text{absolute gain} = G = 10^{(g/10)}$$

$$G = 10^{(35/10)}$$

$$G = 3162$$

Safe Distance – Antenna

$$r = \left[\frac{PG}{4\pi EL}\right]^{1/2}$$

Where:

r is the distance at which the maximum exposure level is exceeded, expressed as (cm).

P is the power emitted, expressed as (mW).

G is absolute gain, a ratio of actual to theoretical power density (dimensionless).

EL is the exposure limit (mW/cm^2).

Use:

To calculate a distance at which the allowable exposure limit is exceeded. Used as a guide for barrier and warning signs.

Example:

The exposure limit is expressed as the power density, which in this case is 10 mW/cm^2. The antenna has a gain of 30 dB and an emitted power of 5000W. You are to post warning signs at the distance at which the EL is reached. How far (in feet) from the antenna should you place your warning signs?

$$r = \left[\frac{PG}{4\pi EL}\right]^{1/2}$$

Step 1: Convert your emitted power from W to mW

$$5000W \times \frac{1000mW}{W} = 5,000,000mW$$

Step 2: Calculate absolute gain

$$\text{Absolute gain} = G = 10^{30/10} = 1000$$

Step 3: Solve for r.

$$r = \left[\frac{(5,000,000mW \times 1000)}{4\pi 10\frac{mW}{cm^2}}\right]^{1/2}$$

$$r = 39,789,909 \; cm$$

Step 4: Convert cm to feet

$$39,789,909 \; cm \times \frac{1 \, ft}{30.48 \, cm} = 1305443 \; ft$$

Exposure Time Allowed – Antenna

$$t = \frac{EL}{ML} \, x \, 0.1h$$

Where:
EL is the exposure limit, expressed as (mW/cm^2).
ML is the measured energy level, expressed as (mW/cm^2).
0.1h is the 6-minute averaging time factor.
t is the maximum acceptable time duration for exposure, expressed as minutes.
Use: To calculate an acceptable exposure time for situations where the exposure exceeds allowed 6-minute exposure limit.
Note: The 6-minute averaging is based on cooling time experimental data for microwave-irradiated animals.

Example:
A worker must work near an antenna with a measured exposure level of 22 mW/cm^2. The exposure limit is 10 mW/cm^2. Calculate the acceptable exposure duration.

$$t = \frac{EL}{ML} \, x \, 0.1h$$

$$t = \frac{10 mW/cm^2}{22 mW/cm^2} \, x \, 0.1 \, h$$

t = 0.045 hours or 2.7 minutes

Note: When given a choice for exposure duration, round down to avoid over exposure.

LASER EQUATIONS

Nominal Hazard Zone – Eye Safe Distance Direct (Intrabeam) Viewing

$$r_{nhz} = \frac{1}{\emptyset}\left[\left(\frac{4\Phi}{\pi EL}\right) - a^2\right]^{1/2}$$

Where:

r_{nhz} is the nominal hazard zone, the area around a laser in which the beam intensity exceeds the exposure limit, expressed as (cm).

$\emptyset$ is the divergence of the emergent light, expressed as radians.

Φ is the total radiant power, expressed as (W).

EL is the exposure limit, expressed as either (mW/cm^2 or J/cm^2).

a is the diameter of the emergent beam, expressed as (cm).

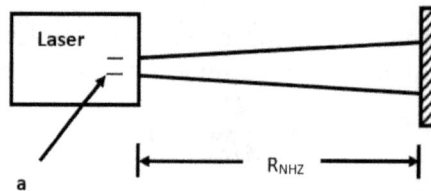

Example:

The laboratory uses a 0.1 W laser, with a beam divergence of 1 mrad and emergent beam diameter of 0.7 cm. The exposure limit is 5×10^{-7} W/cm^2. Calculate the nominal hazard zone distance in feet.

Step 1: Convert milliradians to radians

$$1 \text{ mrad} \times \frac{1\, radian}{1000\, mrad} = .001 \text{ radians}$$

Step 2: Solve for the nominal hazard zone

$$r_{nhz} = \frac{1}{\emptyset}\left[\left(\frac{4\Phi}{\pi EL}\right) - a^2\right]^{1/2}$$

$$r_{nhz} = \frac{1}{.001}\left[\left(\frac{4(0.1)}{\pi(5\, x\, 10^{-7})}\right) - 0.7^2\right]^{1/2}$$

$$r_{nhz} = 504626 \text{ cm}$$

Step 3: Convert centimeters to feet $504626 \text{ cm} \times \frac{1\, foot}{30.48\, cm} = 16{,}555 \text{ feet}$

Nominal Hazard Zone – Eye Safe Distance 'Lens on Laser' Viewing

$$r_{nhz} = \frac{f_0}{b_0}\left(\frac{4\Phi}{\pi EL}\right)^{1/2}$$

Where:

r_{nhz} is the nominal hazard zone, the area around a laser in which the beam intensity exceeds the exposure limit, expressed as (cm).

f_0 is the lens focal length, expressed as (cm).

b_0 is the diameter of the laser beam when focused on the lens, expressed as (cm).

Φ is the total radiant power, expressed as (W).

EL is the exposure limit (aka: MPE), expressed as (W/cm^2).

Use: To calculate the distance from the laser to a point where eye exposure no longer exceeds the exposure limit for lasers equipped with a lens. Safe viewing distance.

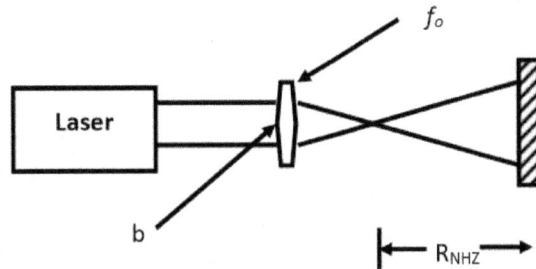

Example:

A laser cutting operation utilizes a 1000 W laser equipped with a 200 mm focal length lens. The laser has a beam size at the lens of 30 mm. The exposure limit is 0.1 W/cm^2. Calculate the nominal hazard zone.

Step 1: Convert millimeters to centimeters

$$200 \text{ mm x } 1\,\frac{1\,cm}{10\,mm} = 20 \text{ cm}$$

$$30 \text{ mm x } 1\,\frac{1\,cm}{10\,mm} = 3 \text{ cm}$$

Step 2: Solve for r_{nhz}

$$r_{nhz} = \frac{f_0}{b_0}\left(\frac{4\Phi}{\pi EL}\right)^{1/2}$$

$$r_{nhz} = \frac{20}{3}\left(\frac{4(1000)}{\pi(0.1)}\right)^{1/2}$$

$$r_{nhz} = 752\ cm\ or\ 7.5\ m$$

$$r_{nhz} = \left(\frac{\rho\Phi\cos\theta}{\pi EL}\right)^{1/2}$$

Where:

r_{nhz} is the nominal hazard zone, the area around a laser in which the beam intensity exceeds the exposure limit, expressed as (cm).

p is reflectivity. The worst case for reflectivity is 100%.

Φ is the total radiant power, expressed as (W).

θ is the viewing angle, expressed as degrees.

EL is the exposure limit (aka: MPE), expressed as (W/cm^2).

Use: To calculate the distance from the laser to a point where eye exposure no longer exceeds the exposure limit for diffuse reflections of the beam from a Lambertian surface. Safe viewing distance.

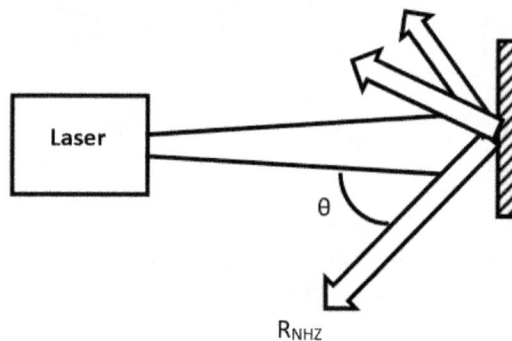

Example:

A 1000 W laser beam is reflecting at a viewing angle of 20 degrees. The surface reflectivity is considered worst case. The exposure limit is 0.1 W/cm^2. Calculate the nominal hazard zone.

$$r_{nhz} = \left(\frac{\rho\Phi\cos\theta}{\pi EL}\right)^{1/2}$$

$$r_{nhz} = \left(\frac{1(1000\cos 20)}{\pi(0.1)}\right)^{1/2}$$

$$r_{nhz} = 54.7 \text{ cm}$$

Acceptable Distance for a Laser Barrier

$$D_s = \frac{1}{\emptyset}\left[\left(\frac{4\Phi}{\pi TL}\right) - a^2\right]^{1/2}$$

Where:

D_s is the separation distance required to provide adequate protection from beam (cm).

$\emptyset$ is the divergence of the emergent light, expressed as radians.

Φ is the total radiant power, expressed as (W).

TL is the threshold limit value of the barrier (mW/cm^2).

a is the diameter of the emergent beam, expressed as (cm).

Use: Calculation of the minimum distance (or installation distance) for a barrier to be sufficiently protective. Barriers placed less than this distance are subject to beam penetration.

Note: This formula is very similar to the nominal hazard zone formula for intra-beam viewing, substituting barrier threshold limit for exposure limit.

Example:

The barrier material has a Threshold Limit of 20 W/cm^2 for 8-hours (worst-case rating). A 250 W laser has a beam divergence of 2 milliradians and an emergent beam diameter of 0.5 cm. Calculate the minimum separation distance.

Step 1: Convert the milliradians to radians

$$2 \text{ mrad} \times \frac{1\,radian}{1000\,mrads} = 0.002 \text{ radians}$$

Step 2: Solve for D_s

$$D_s = \frac{1}{\emptyset}\left[\left(\frac{4\Phi}{\pi TL}\right) - a^2\right]^{1/2}$$

$$D_s = \frac{1}{0.002}\left[\left(\frac{4(250)}{\pi(20)}\right) - 0.5^2\right]^{1/2}$$

$$D_s = 1979 \text{ cm or } 19.8 \text{ m}$$

Note: When given a choice for a barrier, round up to ensure adequate protection.

Laser Beam Diameter

$$D_L = \sqrt{(a^2 + \emptyset^2 r^2)}$$

Where:

D_L is the laser beam diameter at distance or range, expressed as (cm).

a is the emergent beam diameter (cm).

$\emptyset$ is the divergence of the emergent light, expressed as radians.

r is the range or distance, expressed as (cm).

Use: Typically, outdoor uses such as military ranging. The beam diameter is important for eye safety when determining what portion of the beam will enter the pupil. It can also be used in calculating diffuse reflection hazards.

Example:

Calculate the beam diameter at 5 km for a laser range finder. The emergent beam diameter is 2 centimeters, and the beam divergence is 0.1 milliradians.

Step 1: Convert milliradians to radians

$$0.1 \text{ milliradians x } \frac{1\ radian}{1000\ miliiradians} = 0.0001 \text{ radians}$$

Step 2: Convert kilometers to centimeters

$$5 \text{ kilometers x } \frac{100000\ cm}{1\ kilometer} = 500{,}000 \text{ cm}$$

Step 3: Solve for D_L

$$D_L = \sqrt{(a^2 + \emptyset^2 r^2)}$$

$$D_L = \sqrt{(2^2 + (0.0001^2 x 500{,}000^2))}$$

$$D_L = 50 \text{ cm}$$

Rubric 14: Non-Ionizing Radiation Questions

1. What are the two general types of lasers?

    A) Steady beam laser and high frequency laser.
    B) High frequency laser and low frequency laser.
    C) Low frequency laser and pulsed laser.
    D) Steady beam laser and pulsed laser.

2. How would you define a CW laser?

    A) A laser that emits radiation for a time less than 0.25 seconds.
    B) A laser that emits radiation for a time greater than or equal to 0.25 seconds.
    C) A laser that promotes a human aversion response to UV radiation.
    D) A laser that promotes a human aversion response to IR radiation.

3. What type of pulsed laser(s) produces pulses in the picosecond domain?

    A) Q-switched
    B) Mode-locked
    C) Normal pulse
    D) High pulse

4. What are the primary factors in determining the laser hazard level for continuous lasers?

    A) Total energy per pulse and exposure duration.
    B) Average power and radiant exposure.
    C) Average power and exposure duration.
    D) Total energy per pulse and radiant exposure.

5. Acute skin effects of exposure to UV in the 300 nm wavelength range include which of the following?

    A) Erythema, photosensitization.
    B) Melanosome expectoration.
    C) Premature aging.
    D) Hair movement, shock, burns.

6. A worker is exposed to UV radiation for an entire work shift. Which of the following is a dose-dependent inflammation of the corneal tissue?

    A) Conjunctivitis
    B) Photokeratitis
    C) Optical neuritis
    D) Aphakia

7. Which of the following best describes the mechanisms by which laser radiation may produce damage (injury)?

    A) Erythema.
    B) Elastosis, melanosis.
    C) Photomechanical, thermal, photochemical.
    D) Biochemical, pseudoaphakic degradation.

8. Exposure limits (ACGIH) for static magnetic fields are given for whole body general, whole body special, limbs and medical device wearers. What unit is used to define the exposure limit?

    A) Tesla
    B) Roentgen
    C) Curie
    D) SAR

9. The Threshold Limit Value (TLV) for Light and Near Infrared is divided into 4 sections based on potential health effects and spectral regions. Which of the following is not a health effect and spectral region section?

    A) To protect against thermal injury to the cornea and lens from IR.
    B) To protect against retinal photo-chemical injury from chronic blue light.
    C) To protect against macular injury from IR.
    D) To protect against retinal thermal injury from near IR.

10. "Arc eye" or "welder's flash" is a result from high-intensity exposure to UV-B and UV-C. This injury results from exposure of the unprotected eye to a welding arc or other artificial source that is rich in UV-B and UV-C. What is the medical condition for "arc eye" or "welder's flash?"

    A) Photokeratitis and photoconjunctivitis.
    B) Traumatic iritis.
    C) Corneal abrasion.
    D) Subconjunctival hemorrhage.

11. Choose the answer that correctly lists the reason why visual performance in workers over 40 years of age tends to become worse with time.

    A) Pupils decrease in size (Senile Myosis), and fluorescence of the lens.
    B) Loss of accommodation (Presbyopia), and fluorescence of the lens.
    C) Pupils decrease in size (Senile Myosis).
    D) Loss of accommodation (Presbyopia), pupils decrease in size (Senile Myosis), and Fluorescence of the lens.

12. The damage to skin from IR exposure results from a temperature increase in the absorbing tissue. The temperature increase is due to a variety of factors. The factors are:

    A) Wavelength, parameters involved in heat conduction and dissipation, intensity of the exposure, and exposure duration.
    B) Parameters involved in heat conduction and dissipation, intensity of the exposure, and exposure duration.
    C) Wavelength, intensity of the exposure, and exposure duration.
    D) Wavelength and exposure duration.

13. Which of the following is not considered a use of UV radiation?

    A) Photoluminescence.
    B) Treating skin disorders.
    C) Change the channel on a television.
    D) Germicidal applications.

14. Major sources for visible radiation include the sun, various lamps, projection systems, welding arcs, and lasers. If the luminance of the noonday sun is 1.6×10^5 cd/cm, how long will it take for a blue-light injury to occur?

    A) 30 seconds.
    B) 90 seconds.
    C) 180 seconds.
    D) 240 seconds.

15. Key characteristics of light sources are efficiency, color rendering index, and color temperature. Choose the answer below that correctly defines efficiency in relation to light sources.

    A) A relative scale that rates how perceived colors of objects, illuminated by a given source, matches the color produced by the same object when illuminated by a reference standard light source.
    B) The ability of converting energy to visible light.
    C) The ability of converting visible light to energy.
    D) The color of a blackbody radiator at a given temperature.

16. The TLV for retinal injury from light depends on a variety of factors. Which of the following factors listed below is not necessary when dealing with retinal injury from light?

    A) The measured value of spectral radiance.
    B) The viewing duration and angular subtense.
    C) The intensity of light emitted.
    D) The retinal thermal hazard function.

17. Which organization listed below is the proper source to find information on appropriate light levels in an industrial setting?

    A) Industrial Illuminating Administration (IIA).
    B) Illuminating Engineering Society of North America (IESNA).
    C) Illuminating Society for Industrial Engineers (ISIE).
    D) Department of Illuminating Engineering (DIE).

18. Metals, plastics and glasses are efficient barrier or enclosure materials to protect workers from UV exposure. Transmission curves of various filter materials and UV inhibitors are available. Which of the following materials listed below is not useful for UV exposure?

    A) Cellulose Acetate.
    B) Activated Carbon.
    C) Polyester films.
    D) Acrylics.

19. Welding curtains may be made of materials that are either opaque or transparent to visible wavelengths. Choose the answer that correctly states why transparent welding curtains are utilized in an industrial setting.

    A) Allows easier communication with employees and management can keep an eye on employees.
    B) Increases productivity and allows visual contact with welders.
    C) Lowers the airborne concentration of welding fumes and provides an increase of general illumination levels.
    D) Allows visual contact with welders, reduces arc glare, and increases general illumination levels.

20. Example Laser Problem: What is the minimal Optical Density (OD) required of protective eyewear?

    Given:
    ML (Measured Level) = 128 mW/cm^2
    EL (Exposure Limit) = 0.0190 mW/cm^2

    A) 3.83
    B) 4.78
    C) 9.50
    D) 12.78

Rubric 14: Non-Ionizing Radiation Answers

1. Answer: D
Explanation: There are two general types of lasers. The first type of laser generates a continuous wave of light that is emitted as a steady beam. This type of laser has a peak power equal to the average power output, and the beam irradiance is constant with time. Continuous-wave (CW) lasers emit a "temporally constant power of laser light." The second type of laser is the pulsed laser. The pulsed laser has a mode of operation that consists of the emission of either a single pulse, or a series of laser pulses, with pulse periods ranging from a few picoseconds to seconds. Pulsed lasers may be normal pulse, Q-switched, or mode-locked. *Source: The Occupational Environment: Its Evaluation, Control and Management 3rd Edition, Volume 2*

2. Answer: B
Explanation: For a frame of reference, consider that the innate human aversion response time to bright light, including invisible laser light, is approximately 0.25 seconds. Note that the aversion response does not occur with exposure to invisible radiation such as UV and IR. If a laser emits radiation for a time greater than or equal to 0.25 seconds, it is defined as a continuous-wave (CW) laser. *Source: The Occupational Environment: Its Evaluation, Control and Management 3rd Edition, Volume 2*

3. Answer: B
Explanation: Pulse widths should be much shorter than the aversion response time. These are realized with Q-switched or mode locked pulses. Q-switching produces pulses on the order of a few nanoseconds to microseconds, while mode-locked pulses are even shorter, in the picosecond domain. Special pulsing techniques, such as cavity dumping, can produce pulses in approximately femtoseconds. *Source: The Occupational Environment: Its Evaluation, Control and Management 3rd Edition, Volume 2*

4. Answer: C
Explanation: For continuous lasers, the average power and exposure duration are the primary factors in determining the laser hazard level. To evaluate pulsed laser safety, the following items must be considered: total energy per pulse, peak power, pulse duration, pulse repetition, frequency, and radiant exposure. *Source: The Occupational Environment: Its Evaluation, Control and Management 3rd Edition, Volume 2*

5. Answer: A
Explanation: The penetration depth of UV into tissue is dependent on wavelength, tissue thickness, and pigmentation (melanin). Wavelengths less than 300 nm are primarily absorbed in the epidermis, while wavelengths longer than 297 nm penetrate into the dermis. Erythema is reddening of the skin and photosensitization is an abnormal skin reaction to UV in the presence of a chemical. Penetration is greater in fair skin than dark. *Source: Applications and Computational Elements of Industrial Hygiene, Stern and Mansdorf.*

6. Answer: B

Explanation: Conjunctivitis is inflammation of the conjunctiva. Aphakia is a condition in which the lens of the eye is missing. Photokeratitis is inflammation of the cornea. Cataracts are also related to UV exposure. *Source: Applications and Computational Elements of Industrial Hygiene, Stern and Mansdorf.*

7. Answer: C

Explanation: There are three ways that laser radiation may produce damage: 1) Photomechanical, 2) Thermal, and 3) Photochemical. Photomechanical effects are related to brief pulses of extremely high levels of irradiance that can damage tissues. Thermal effects occur when radiant energy is absorbed, heating and damaging tissue. Photochemical effects are related to the UV laser exposure, as well as exposure to blue and green light. Exposure to UV laser can cause DNA damage. *Source: Applications and Computational Elements of Industrial Hygiene, Stern and Mansdorf.*

8. Answer: A

Explanation:

TLV for Static Magnetic Fields 2015

Exposure	Ceiling Value
Whole Body (general workplace)	2 Tesla
Whole Body (special worker training and controlled work-place environment)	8 Tesla
Medical device wearers	0.5 Tesla
Limbs	20 Tesla

Note: Tesla is abbreviated as T.

9. Answer: C

Explanation: The four sections: To protect against thermal injury to the cornea and lens from IR, to protect against retinal photo-chemical injury from chronic blue light, to protect against retinal thermal injury from near IR, and to protect against retinal thermal injury from a visible light source. *Source: ACGIH Threshold Limit Values for Chemical Substances and Physical Agents 2015.*

10. Answer: A

Explanation: UV-B and UV-C are primarily absorbed in the tissue of the cornea and conjunctiva. Corneal transmission ranges from 60% to 83% in the UV-A band, with much of the energy absorbed by the lens. Photokeratitis and photoconjunctivitis result from acute, high-intensity exposure to UV-B and UV-C. Commonly referred to as "arc eye" or "welder's flash" by workers, this injury results from exposure of the unprotected eye to a welding arc or other artificial sources rich in UV-B and UV-C. Sunlight exposure produces these sequelae only in environments where highly reflective materials are present, such as snow (snow blindness) or sand. *Source: The Occupational Environment: Its Evaluation, Control, and Management 3rd Edition Volume 2*

11. Answer: D

Explanation: There are several reasons why visual performance in workers over 40 years of age tends to become worse with time. A loss of accommodation around 40-45 years of age makes it harder to focus at short working distances. This phenomenon is known as presbyopia. The pupils become smaller with age (senile myosis). The amount of light reaching the retina is reduced due to absorption of shorter wavelengths in the lens and increased scatter of the light entering the eye. The optical density of the lens increases mainly to effects of UV radiation on the lens. Finally, the lens starts to fluoresce due to aging factors. The net result is reduced visual acuity; contrast sensitivity; color discrimination; and increased sensitivity to glare, which requires longer periods of recovery from exposure to high luminance fields. *Source: The Occupational Environment: Its Evaluation, Control, and Management 3rd Edition Volume 2*

12. Answer: A

Explanation: The damage to skin from IR exposure results from a temperature increase in the absorbing tissue. The increase depends on the wavelength, the parameters involved in heat conduction and dissipation, the intensity of the exposure, and the exposure duration. The most prominent effects near-IR include acute skin burn, increased vasodilation of the capillary beds, and an increased pigmentation that can persists for long periods of time. With continuous exposure to high-intensity IR, the erythematous appearance due to vasodilation may become permanent. *Source: The Occupational Environment: Its Evaluation, Control, and Management 3rd Edition Volume 2*

13. Answer: C

Explanation: UV radiation uses include curing materials; sun tanning; photoluminescence; chemical manufacturing; treating skin disorders; germicidal applications; UV spectroscopy; and photomicrolithography. *Source: The Occupational Environment: Its Evaluation, Control, and Management 3rd Edition Volume 2*

14. Answer: B

Explanation: The sun is the major source for visible radiation, along with lamps, projection systems, welding arcs, and lasers. The luminance of the noonday sun is 1.6×10^5 cd/cm, while the time necessary for blue-light injury is about 90 seconds. Xenon short-arc lamps emit relatively high levels of blue light, while low-pressure fluorescent lamps emit relatively low levels. Luminance levels for xenon short-arc lamps were around 10^4 to 10^5 cd/cm. *Source: The Occupational Environment: Its Evaluation, Control, and Management 3rd Edition Volume 2*

15. Answer: B

Explanation: Key characteristics of light sources are efficiency, color rendering index, and color temperature.
Efficiency – The ability to convert energy to visible light.
Color Rendering Index – A relative scale that rates how perceived colors of objects illuminated by a given source match the color produced by the same object when illuminated by a reference standard light source.
Color Temperature – The color of a blackbody radiator at a given temperature. *Source: The Occupational Environment: Its Evaluation, Control, and Management 3rd Edition Volume 2*

16. Answer: C

Explanation: ACGIH has recommended criteria for source luminance (1 cd/cm2); retinal thermal injury from visible light; retinal photochemical from blue light; retinal thermal injury from IR-A; and corneal and lenticular injury from IR-A and IR-B radiation. TLV for retinal injury from light depends upon the measured value of spectral radiance; the viewing duration; the angular subtense; and a weighting factor called the retinal thermal hazard function [R(λ)]. *Source: The Occupational Environment: Its Evaluation, Control, and Management 3rd Edition Volume 2*

17. Answer: B

Explanation: Current information about appropriate light levels are available from the Illuminating Engineering Society of North America (IESNA). The IESNA has established a generalized procedure to aid in selecting the necessary illuminance based on knowledge of space, task, and occupant characteristics. In the IESNA handbook, there are seven illuminance section criteria, which are divided into three visual task groups: simple, common, and special. *Source: The Occupational Environment: Its Evaluation, Control, and Management 3rd Edition Volume 2*

18. Answer: B

Explanation: Barriers or enclosures are comprised of efficient attenuating materials, including metals, plastics, and glasses. Transmission curves of various filter materials and UV inhibitors are available. Some useful UV filter materials are polyester films, cellulose acetate, and acrylics, such as methyl methacrylate based polymers. *Source: The Occupational Environment: Its Evaluation, Control, and Management 3rd Edition Volume 2*

19. Answer: D

Explanation: Commercially available welding curtains are comprised of materials that are either opaque or transparent to visible wavelengths. Opaque materials include canvas duck, asbestos substitutes, and polymer laminates. Transparent welding curtains may allow visual contact with welders, reduce arc glare, and increase general illumination levels. *Source: The Occupational Environment: Its Evaluation, Control, and Management 3rd Edition Volume 2*

20. Answer: A

Explanation:

$$O.D._{needed} = \log\left[\frac{ML}{EL}\right] = \log\left[\frac{128 \text{ mW/cm}^2}{0.0190 \text{ mW/cm}^2}\right] = \log[6737] = 3.83$$

Source: University of Utah

Rubric 15: Thermal Stressors

A commonly encountered occupational exposure is adverse thermal environments. Workers can experience physiological stress from thermal stressors, such as hot and cold environments. Protection from the stressors requires recognition of potential problems, minimization of heat or cool strain, and determination of the most practical and effective solutions. This is achieved by providing guidance to workers and supervisors to understand the fundamentals of worker thermoregulation and exposure control.

Important Terms and Concepts

Acclimatization- Adaptation of a species or a population to a changed environment over several generations.

Corrected effective temperature- An index of thermal stress similar to the effective temperature index; however, globe temperature is used instead of dry bulb temperature.

Dew point temperature- (1) The temperature and pressure at which a gas begins to condense to a liquid. (2) The temperature at which air becomes saturated when cooled without addition of moisture or change of pressure; any further cooling causes condensation.

Hygrometer- An instrument to measure humidity in the atmosphere.

Hyponatremia- Subnormal or reduced blood sodium levels.

Hypotonic- Referring to a solution with a lower osmotic pressure than physiological saline.

Mean radiant temperature- The mean radiant temperature is the temperature of an imaginary black enclosure of uniform wall temperature, which provides the same radiant heat loss of gain as the environment measured. It can be approximated from readings of globe temperature, dry bulb temperature, and air velocity.

Metabolic heat- Heat generated by the body's physical and chemical processes.

Psychrometer- An instrument consisting of wet and dry bulb thermometers for measuring relative humidity.

Relative humidity- The ratio of the quantity of water vapor present in the air to the quantity that would saturate it at any specific temperature.

Thermal balance- The heat exchange between the human body and the environment.

Heat strain disorder protection requires anticipating problems and trying to prevent and mitigate disorders from developing. Important defensive measures include gradually acclimatizing workers, keeping workers well hydrated, and detecting symptoms of heat strain.

Heat Illness- First Aid Treatment and Signs and Symptoms

Heat Illness	First Aid Treatment	Signs and Symptoms
Heat cramps	Salted fluids by mouth, or IV infusion.	Painful spasms of muscles used during work. Onset during or after work hours.
Heat exhaustion	Remove to cooler environment, rest in a reclined position, administer fluids. Rest until rehydrated.	Fatigue, nausea, headache, giddiness. Skin clammy and pale.
Heat Stroke	Immediate and rapid cooling by immersion in chilled water with massage or by wrapping in wet sheet with vigorous fanning. Medical attention needed.	Hot, dry skin. Rectal temperature above 40.5°C. Confusion, loss of consciousness, convulsions.

An effective temperature index combines air temperature, humidity and air movement to produce a single index termed an effective temperature. Another index is the wet bulb globe temperature (WBGT). The WBGT combines the effect of four (4) thermal components affecting heat stress: air temperature, humidity, air velocity, and radiant heat, as measured by the dry bulb, natural wet bulb, and globe temperatures. Wet bulb temperature is the temperature as determined by the wet bulb thermometer or a standard sling psychrometer, or its equivalent. This temperature is influenced by the evaporation rate of the water, which in turn depends on the humidity (amount of water vapor) in the air. A wet bulb thermometer is a thermometer with the bulb covered by a cloth saturated with water. The dry bulb temperature is the temperature of air as determined by a standard thermometer. Temperature units are expressed in degrees Celsius, Kelvin, or Fahrenheit. Globe temperature is the measure of radiant heat. *Source: The Occupational Environment: Its Evaluation, Control, and Management, 3rd Ed. and Fundamentals of Industrial Hygiene, 5th Edition*

Cold stress is another thermal hazard to workers. The first psychological response to cold stress is to conserve body heat by reducing blood circulation through the skin. The most significant effect of cold exposure is on manual dexterity. Many studies of performance in cold emphasized the effects of cold on the skillful use of the hands. Another physiological response is shivering. Shivering increases the rate of metabolism and is a good sign that the cold stress is significant and that hypothermia may be present. The primary response to preventing excessive exposure to cold stress is human behavior. Behaviors include increasing clothing insulation, increasing activity, and seeking warm locations. See the table below of cold-related disorders including the symptoms, signs and causes.

Cold-Related Disorders

Disorder	Causes	Signs	Symptoms
Raynaud's Disorder	Exposure to cold. Exposure to vibration. Vascular disease.	Fingers blanch with cold exposure.	Fingers tingle. Intermittent blanching and reddening.
Chilblain	Inadequate clothing. Exposure to cold and dampness. Vascular disease.	Swelling. Severe spasms.	Recurrent localized itching. Painful inflammation.
Trench Foot	Exposure to cold (above freezing). Dampness.	Edema. Blisters. Response to touch depends on depth of freezing.	Severe pain. Tingling. Itching.
Frostnip	Exposure to cold (above freezing).	Skin turns white.	Possible itching or pain.
Frostbite	Exposure to cold. Vascular disease.	Skin color white or grayish, then yellow, reddish violet, to black. Blisters. Response to touch depends on depth of freezing.	Burning sensation at first followed by coldness, numbness, and tingling.
Hypothermia	Excessive exposure to low temperatures. Exhaustion or dehydration. Abnormal tolerance (genetic or acquired). Drug/alcohol use.	Euphoria. Slowed and weak pulse. Slurred speech. Shivering, loss of consciousness with body temperature < 95 F.	Chills. Pain in extremities. Fatigue or drowsiness.

Formulas and Calculations

WBGT with Solar Load (Outdoors)

$$WBGT = 0.7t_{nwb} + 0.2t_g + 0.1t_{db}$$

Where:

WBGT is the wet bulb globe temperature, expressed as either Fahrenheit or Celsius

t_{nwb} is the natural wet bulb temperature, expressed as Fahrenheit or Celsius

t_g is the globe temperature, expressed as Fahrenheit or Celsius

t_{db} is the dry bulb temperature, expressed as Fahrenheit or Celsius

Use: The calculation can be used to determine the risk of heat stress based on the Wet Bulb Globe Temperature (WBGT) Index.

Note: The formula is for use outside on a sunny day.

Example:

Calculate the WBGT reading for paving contractors at a construction worksite. There is no shade and the work is in full sun. The WBGT readings are as follows: the natural wet bulb measures 84°F, the globe temperature is 97°F, and the dry bulb temperature is 92°F?

$$WBGT = 0.7t_{nwb} + 0.2t_g + 0.1t_{db}$$

$$t_{nwb} = 84°F$$
$$t_g = 97°F$$
$$t_{db} = 92°F$$

Step 1: Solve for WBGT

$$WBGT = 0.7(84) + 0.2(97) + 0.1(92)$$

$$WBGT = 87°F$$

WBGT Without Solar Load (Indoor, Cloudy, Night)

$$WBGT = 0.7t_{nwb} + 0.3t_g$$

Where:

WBGT is the wet bulb globe temperature, expressed as Fahrenheit or Celsius

t_{nwb} is the natural wet bulb temperature, expressed as Fahrenheit or Celsius

t_g is the globe temperature, expressed as Fahrenheit or Celsius

Use: The calculation can be used to determine the risk of heat stress based on the Wet Bulb Globe Temperature (WBGT) Index.

Note: The formula is for use indoors, or for outside when not in the sun

Example:

Calculate the WBGT index for work inside an industrial rmanufacturing facility. The WBGT provides the following readings: the natural wet bulb temperature measures 81°F and the globe temperature is 95°F.

$$WBGT = 0.7t_{nwb} + 0.3t_g$$

$$t_{nwb} = 81°F$$
$$t_g = 95°F$$

Step 1: Calculate the WBGT

$$WBGT = 0.7(81) + 0.3(95)$$

$$WBGT = 85°F$$

Heat Storage by Body

$$\Delta S = (M - W) \pm C \pm R - E$$

Where:

ΔS is the change in amount of heat stored by the body expressed as kcal/hr; BTU/hr

M is the metabolic heat, expressed as kcal/hr; BTU/hr

W is the external work rate, expressed as kcal/hr; BTU/hr

C is the convective heat loss/gain from air movement, expressed as kcal/hr; BTU/hr

R is the radiant heat loss/gain, expressed as kcal/hr; BTU/hr

E is the evaporative heat loss, expressed as kcal/hr; BTU/hr

Use: Describes the change in the body heat load associated the exchange of heat between the body and the environment.

Example:

Calculate the change in body heat level for a worker who is has a workload of $1500\frac{BTU}{hr}$. The conditions are: 1) convective heat gain is $50\frac{BTU}{hr}$, 2) the radiant heat gain is $70\frac{BTU}{hr}$, and 3) the evaporative heat loss is $500\frac{BTU}{hr}$?

$$\Delta S = (M - W) \pm C \pm R - E$$

$$M - W = 1500\,\frac{BTU}{hr}$$

$$C = 50\,\frac{BTU}{hr}$$

$$R = 70\,\frac{BTU}{hr}$$

$$E = 500\frac{BTU}{hr}$$

Step 1: Solve for ΔS

$$\Delta S = \left(1500\,\frac{BTU}{hr}\right) + \left(50\,\frac{BTU}{hr}\right) + \left(70\,\frac{BTU}{hr}\right) - \left(500\,\frac{BTU}{hr}\right)$$

$$\Delta S = 1120\,\frac{BTU}{hr}$$

The Heat Stress Index

$$HSI = \frac{E_{req}}{E_{max}} \; x \; 100$$

Where:

HSI is the heat stress index, expressed as a percentage (i.e. the value x 100)

E_{req} is the amount of evaporative heat necessary to prevent heat stress, expressed as kcal/hr; BTU/hr

E_{max} is the maximum evaporative heat loss for the existing conditions, expressed as kcal/hr; BTU/hr

Use: To calculate the amount of evaporative heat loss necessary to maintain thermal balance.

Note: An HSI value of zero indicates no heat stress, and a value up to 100% is predicted to be tolerated by the fit and acclimatized.

Example:

The facility subject matter expert informs you that the required evaporative heat loss is $3{,}000 \frac{BTU}{hr}$ and the maximum evaporative heat loss is $3{,}500 \frac{BTU}{hr}$. Calculate the heat stress index.

$$HSI = \frac{E_{req}}{E_{max}} \; x \; 100$$

$$E_{req} = 3{,}000 \frac{BTU}{hr}$$
$$E_{max} = 3{,}500 \frac{BTU}{hr}$$

Step 1: Solve for HSI

$$HSI = \frac{3{,}000}{3{,}500} \; x \; 100$$

$$HSI = 86\%$$

Rubric 15: Thermal Stressors Questions

1. Which of the following best describes conduction?

   A) The transfer of heat between two objects using electromagnetic radiation.
   B) The transfer of heat by air movement or air currents.
   C) The transfer of heat from cooler to warmer objects.
   D) The transfer of heat when two objects come into contact.

2. Which of the following lists the primary methods of heat transfer?

   A) Radiation, convection, conduction.
   B) Hot to cold objects.
   C) Evaporation, condensation.
   D) Solar, desalinization.

3. What condition is characterized by red papules in areas where clothing contacts skin, and may be caused by excess sweat absorbed by the keratinous layer of the skin?

   A) Heat cramps.
   B) Measles.
   C) Prickly heat.
   D) Rocky Mountain Spotted Fever.

4. Normal body functioning is maintained, in part, by the body's ability to maintain a relatively constant core temperature. Heat is generated internally by metabolic activity. Which part of the central nervous system is responsible for thermoregulation in humans?

   A) Heat cramps.
   B) Medulla oblongata.
   C) Cerebellum.
   D) Hypothalamus.

5. What are the primary determinants in cold related injury?

   A) Radiant temperature and relative humidity.
   B) Relative humidity and wind speed.
   C) Air temperature and wind speed.
   D) Air temperature and radiant temperature.

6. The primary method for cooling of the human body is:

   A) Resting.
   B) Evaporation.
   C) Convection.
   D) Radiation.

7. How can monitoring the heart rate of workers be helpful in preventing heat stress?

    A) Worker performance and effort can be compared with desired productivity measures.
    B) The heart rate correlates positively with body temperature.
    C) Cardiac fitness models can be integrated into wellness programs.
    D) The heart rate can be used as a surrogate for oxygen consumption as an index of work intensity.

8. A worker is working the night shift on the loading docks in Miami, Florida. The safety technician measures the natural wet bulb = 85°F, and the globe temperature = 84°F. What is the WBGT reading?

    A) 84.7
    B) 87
    C) 169
    D) 91

9. If the work force is performing moderate work (350 kcal/hour), and the WBGT reading is 84.7 F., what is the designated work-rest regimen for an acclimatized worker based on the table shown below?

Work-Rest Regimen	Heavy Work	Moderate Work	Light Work
25% Work 75% Rest	30.0	31.1	32.2
50% Work 50% Rest	27.9	29.4	31.4
75% Work 25% Rest	27.9 25.9	29.4 28.0	30.6
Continuous	25.0	26.7	30.0

    A) 75% work – 25% rest
    B) 50% work – 50% rest
    C) 25% work – 75% rest
    D) Continuous work

10. What are some signs and symptoms of heat exhaustion?

    A) Fatigue, nausea, headache, giddiness. Skin clammy and pale.
    B) Painful spasms of muscles used during work. Onset during or after work hours.
    C) Hot, dry skin. Rectal temperature above 40.5°C. Confusion, loss of consciousness, convulsions.
    D) Miliaria rubra and Miliaria profunda.

11. Using the equation below, calculate the heat stress index for a worker who has a required evaporation of 40 kcal/hour and a maximal evaporation of 100 kcal/hour. Use the evaluation of heat stress index table to determine the physiologic and hygienic implications of 8-hour exposures to heat stress index.

A) -20, Mild cold strain
B) 0, No thermal strain
C) +40, Severe heat strain
D) +70, Very severe heat strain

$$HSI = \left(\frac{E_{req}}{E_{max}}\right) x \ 100$$

Evaluation of Heat Stress Index

Heat Stress Index	PHYSIOLOGIC AND HYGIENIC IMPLICATIONS OF 8-HOUR EXPOSURES TO HEAT STRESS INDEX
+100	• Maximum strain tolerated by fit, acclimatized young workers.
+70	• Very severe heat strain. • Only a small percentage of the population may be expected to qualify for this work. Personnel should be selected (a) by medical examination and (b) by trial on the job (after acclimatization). • Special measures are needed to assure adequate water and salt intake. • Amelioration of work conditions by any feasible means is highly desirable and may be expected to decrease the health hazard, while increasing efficiency on the job. • Slight "indisposition", which in most jobs would be insufficient to affect performance, may render workers unfit for this exposure.
+40	• Severe heat strain involving a threat to health unless workers are physically fit. • Break periods are required for workers not previously acclimatized. • Some decrement in performance of physical work is to be expected. • Medical selection of personnel is desirable because these conditions are unsuitable for those with cardiovascular or respiratory impairments or with chronic dermatitis. • These working conditions are also unsuitable for activities requiring sustained mental effort.
+10	• Mild to moderate heat strain. • For a job that involves higher intellectual function, dexterity, or alertness, subtle to substantial decrements in performance are expected. • In the performance of heavy physical work, little decrement is expected unless the ability of individuals to perform such work under marginal stress would be expected to be detrimental.
0	• No thermal strain.
-20	• Mild cold strain. • This condition frequently exists in areas where recovery from exposures to heat occurs.

12. Assume wind speed is 5.8 m/sec and air temperature is 40°C. Calculate the convective heat exchange.

A) $48.7 \frac{kcal}{hr}$

B) $65.0 \frac{kcal}{hr}$

C) $83.1 \frac{kcal}{hr}$

D) $100.5 \frac{kcal}{hr}$

$$C = 7.0\, V_{air}^{0.6}(t_{air} - t_{skin})$$

Where:
C = Convective heat exchange, kcal/hour
V_{air} = Air velocity, meters per second
t_{air} = Air temperature, °C
t_{skin} = Mean weighted skin temperature (often assumed to be 35°C)

13. What is the work-rest regimen of a worker performing moderate work when the WBGT reading is 29.4°C?

A) Continuous
B) 75% work, 25% rest
C) 50% work, 50% rest
D) 25% work, 75%rest

14. A laborer on a construction site is responsible for lifting concrete blocks that weigh approximately 25 pounds. He performs this lift approximately 10 ten times per minute over the course of his shift. What workload is this considered?

A) Light work.
B) Medium work.
C) Heavy work.
D) Very heavy work.

15. _____ is a physical change that allows the body to adjust to working in the heat over a period of time.

A) Adaptation.
B) Acclimatization.
C) Tolerance.
D) Heat illness prevention program.

16. Which of the following is an effective way to manage heat stress exposure for workers?

A) Schedule the most strenuous jobs early in the day to avoid the hottest part of the day.
B) Reduce the distance between the worker and radiant heat source.
C) Increase employee rest times when temperature increases.
D) All of the above.

17. An employee on a worker rotation is exposed to different work conditions throughout their shift. Assuming the employee is exposed to 32°C for 2 hours, 29ºC for 2 hours, and 25ºC for 4 hours. What is the employee's average WBGT exposure during the shift?

    A) 90°F
    B) 95°F
    C) 82°F
    D) 78°F

18. What OSHA standard addresses heat stress within general industry?

    A) 1910.95
    B) 1910.178
    C) 1910.179
    D) Currently OSHA does not have a Heat Stress Standard

19. Assuming the following conditions, what is the WBGT index for a day shift employee who is working outside for the entire shift?

    - Wet bulb temperature = 26°C
    - Globe temperature = 35°C
    - Dry bulb temperature = 30°C

    A) 28°C
    B) 30°C
    C) 34°C
    D) 38°C

20. Which of the following engineering controls would be the best solution to provide protection against heat stress in an indoor manufacturing environment?

    A) Large fans to increase air movement.
    B) Worker rotation program to limit worker exposure to heat stress.
    C) Dilution ventilation that pulls make-up air from the outside.
    D) Providing employees with cooling vests.

Rubric 15: Thermal Stressors Answers

1. Answer: D

   Explanation: Conduction is the transfer of heat between two objects from the hotter to the colder object. Convection is the transfer of heat by air movement. Radiant heat is the transfer of heat using electromagnetic radiation such as molten metal or the sun making the skin warm. *Source: Applications and Computational Elements of Industrial Hygiene, Stern and Mansdorf*

2. Answer: A

   Explanation: Conduction is the transfer of heat between two objects from the hotter to the colder object. Convection is the transfer of heat by air movement. Radiant heat is the transfer of heat using electromagnetic radiation, such as molten metal or the sun, making the skin warm. *Source: Applications and Computational Elements of Industrial Hygiene, Stern and Mansdorf*

3. Answer: C

   Explanation: Prickly heat is characterized by red papules in areas where clothing contacts skin, and may be caused as excess sweat is absorbed by the keratinous layer of the skin. *Source: Applications and Computational Elements of Industrial Hygiene, Stern and Mansdorf*

4. Answer: D

   Explanation: Through neural transmitters, the hypothalamus is able to sense temperature changes in the skin, muscle, stomach, etc., and signal either heat conserving or heat dissipating mechanisms. *Source: Applications and Computational Elements of Industrial Hygiene, Stern and Mansdorf*

5. Answer: C

   Explanation: A common method for evaluating the potential for skin freezing is the Equivalent Temperature (Wind Chill Index), which was developed by the U.S. Army Research Institute of Environmental Medicine. This method utilizes air temperature and wind speed. Wet clothing, humidity and work rate can have an effect on the outcome of cold exposure and injury, but are not the primary determinants. *Source: Applications and Computational Elements of Industrial Hygiene, Stern and Mansdorf*

6. Answer: B

   Explanation: Evaporation of sweat is the primary method of cooling for humans. Convection via air movement can improve the effectiveness of the evaporative cooling. *Source: Applications and Computational Elements of Industrial Hygiene, Stern and Mansdorf*

7. Answer: D

   Explanation: Oxygen intake is important for maintaining body temperature. The baseline level of oxygen consumption is the resting metabolic rate measure of liters of oxygen per minute. As physical work increases, oxygen consumption increases, and heat released within the body also increases. Each liter of oxygen consumed releases approximately 4.8 kcal of heat energy inside the body. *Source: Applications and Computational Elements of Industrial Hygiene, Stern and Mansdorf*

8. Answer: A

Explanation:

WBGT = 0.7NWB + 0.3GT for indoor or outdoor with no solar load

WBGT = 0.7 x 85 + 0.3 x 84

WBGT = 84.7°F

9. Answer: B

Work-Rest Regimen	Heavy Work	Moderate Work	Light Work
25% Work 75% Rest	30.0	31.1	32.2
50% Work 50% Rest	27.9	29.4	31.4
75% Work 25% Rest	27.9 25.9	29.4 28.0	30.6
Continuous	25.0	26.7	30.0

Explanation:

First you must convert 84.7 °F to °C.   °C = (°F – 32) x 5/9   °C = 29.3

Looking at the table in the moderate work column and determine that 29.3 is between the 75% work temperature and 50% work temperature; therefore, choose the 50% work regimen.

10. Answer: A

Explanation:

Heat Illness- First Aid Treatment and Signs and Symptoms

Heat Illness	First Aid Treatment	Signs and Symptoms
Heat cramps	• Salted fluids by mouth, or IV infusion.	• Painful spasms of muscles used during work. • Onset during or after work hours.
Heat exhaustion	• Remove to cooler environment, rest in a reclined position, and administer fluids. • Rest until rehydrated.	• Fatigue, nausea, headache, giddiness. Skin clammy and pale.
Heat stroke	• Immediate and rapid cooling by immersion in chilled water with massage or by wrapping in wet sheet with vigorous fanning. • Medical attention needed.	• Hot, dry skin. • Rectal temperature above 40.5°C. • Confusion, loss of consciousness, convulsions.

11. Answer: C

Evaluation of Heat Stress Index

Heat Stress Index	PHYSIOLOGIC AND HYGIENIC IMPLICATIONS OF 8-HOUR EXPOSURES TO HEAT STRESS INDEX
+100	• Maximum strain tolerated by fit, acclimatized young workers.
+70	• Very severe heat strain. • Only a small percentage of the population may be expected to qualify for this work. Personnel should be selected (a) by medical examination and (b) by trial on the job (after acclimatization). • Special measures are needed to assure adequate water and salt intake. • Amelioration of work conditions by any feasible means is highly desirable and may be expected to decrease the health hazard, while increasing efficiency on the job. • Slight "indisposition", which in most jobs would be insufficient to affect performance, may render workers unfit for this exposure.
+40	• Severe heat strain involving a threat to health unless workers are physically fit. • Break periods are required for workers not previously acclimatized. • Some decrement in performance of physical work is to be expected. • Medical selection of personnel is desirable because these conditions are unsuitable for those with cardiovascular or respiratory impairments or with chronic dermatitis. • These working conditions are also unsuitable for activities requiring sustained mental effort.
+10	• Mild to moderate heat strain. • For a job that involves higher intellectual function, dexterity, or alertness, subtle to substantial decrements in performance are expected. • In the performance of heavy physical work, little decrement is expected unless the ability of individuals to perform such work under marginal stress would be expected to be detrimental
0	• No thermal strain.
-20	• Mild cold strain. • This condition frequently exists in areas where recovery from exposures to heat occurs.

Explanation:

$$HSI = \left(\frac{E_{req}}{E_{max}}\right) x\ 100$$

$$HSI = \left(\frac{40\ kcal/hour}{100\ kcal/hour}\right) x\ 100$$

$HSI = 40$, Severe heat strain
Source: Applications and Computational Elements of Industrial Hygiene

12. Answer: D

$$C = 7.0\, V_{air}^{0.6}(t_{air} - t_{skin})$$

Where:
C = Convective heat exchange, kcal/hour
V_{air} = Air velocity, meters per second
t_{air} = Air temperature, °C
t_{skin} = Mean weighted skin temperature (often assumed to be 35°C)

Explanation:
One potential source of heat load to the body is heat exchange between the air and skin of a worker. It is a function of air temperature, mean skin temperature, and wind speed.

$$C = 7.0\, V_{air}^{0.6}(t_{air} - t_{skin})$$

$$C = 7.0\,(5.8\frac{m}{sec})^{\,0.6}(40°C - 35°C)$$

$$C = 100.5\frac{kcal}{hr}$$

Source: Applications and Computational Elements of Industrial Hygiene

13. Answer: C
Explanation:
The ACGIH TLV is designed to prevent heat illness in healthy, acclimatized workers. The table shows WBGT limits for work at light, moderate, and heavy workloads.

Heat Stress Threshold Limit Values- WBGT Threshold Limit Values, °C

Work-Rest Regimen	Heavy Work	Moderate Work	Light Work
25% Work 75% Rest	30.0	31.1	32.2
50% Work 50% Rest	27.9	29.4	31.4
75% Work 25% Rest	27.9 25.9	29.4 28.0	30.6
Continuous	25.0	26.7	30.0

14. Answer: C
Explanation: This employee would be exposed to a heavy workload based upon the classification of the work. *Sources: (1) The Occupational Environment, its Evaluation, Control, and Management (S.R. DiNardi, Editor), (2) American Industrial Hygiene Association ACGIH, 2011, (3) Heat Stress and Strain, in TLVs and BEIs, American Conference of Industrial Hygienists, Cincinnati, OH*

15. Answer: B

Explanation: Acclimatization is defined as a physical change that allows the body to build tolerance to working in the heat. It occurs gradually by increasing workloads and heat exposure. It may take up to 14 days to become fully acclimatized. *Source: The Occupational Environment, its Evaluation, Control, and Management (S.R. DiNardi, Editor), American Industrial Hygiene Association*

16. Answer: D

Explanation: All of the answers are effective ways to manage heat stress to the employee. Where possible, it is a good practice to limit work during the afternoon hours since they are generally the hottest period of the day. If the work must be completed during the hottest times of the day, then proper consideration should be given to work rest cycles. *Source: The Occupational Environment, its Evaluation, Control, and Management (S.R. DiNardi, Editor), American Industrial Hygiene Association*

17. Answer: C

Explanation:

Step 1: Determine WBGT Average Temperature

$$WBGT_{AVG} = \frac{WBGT_1 \times T_1 + WBGT_2 \times T_2 + WBGT_n \times T_n}{T_1 + T_2 + T_n}$$

$$WBGT_{AVG} = \frac{(32 \times 2) + (29 \times 2) + (25 \times 4)}{2 + 2 + 4}$$

$$WBGT_{AVG} = \frac{222}{8}$$

$$WBGT_{AVG} = 28°C$$

Step 2: Convert from Celsius to Fahrenheit

$$T_{°F} = T_{°C} \times {}^9\!/_5 + 32$$

$$T_{°F} = \left(28 \times {}^9\!/_5\right) + 32$$

$$T_{°F} = 82°F$$

The employee is exposed to an average WBGT of 82°F. In this two-part question, it was critical to remember to convert from Celsius to Fahrenheit before answering. *Source: The Occupational Environment, its Evaluation, Control, and Management, AIHA*

18. Answer: D

   Explanation: OSHA does not have a standard that deals specifically with heat stress. Citations for heat stress related matters generally come under section 5(a)1 of the Occupational Safety and Health act of 1970, which is better known as the "General Duty Clause."

19. Answer: A

   - Wet bulb temperature = 26°C
   - Globe temperature = 35°C
   - Dry bulb temperature = 30°C

   Explanation: Calculate the WBGT value

   $$WBGT = 0.7 + 0.2GT + 0.1DB$$

   $$WBGT = 0.7 \times 26 + 0.2 \times 35 + 0.1 \times 30$$

   $$WBGT = 28° \ C$$

   Since the employee is working outside for his or her entire shift, solar load (dry bulb temperature) must be utilized. *Source: The Occupational Environment, its Evaluation, Control, and Management, AIHA*

20. Answer: C

   Explanation: Dilution ventilation would be the best solution because it uses cooler outside make up air to replace the hot air in the building. While using large fans is an option in some manufacturing environments, the fans do not address the temperature of the air. Using a worker rotation and providing cooling vests are administrative controls, which will not do anything to address the heat in the manufacturing environment.

Rubric 16: Toxicology

Toxicology is one of the most important scientific disciplines for the practice of occupational hygiene. Occupational toxicology, a sub-specialty of toxicology, focuses on the relationship between workers and exposures to toxic agents; it is a relatively young field that emerged since the works of Alice Hamilton.

The paraphrased words of Paracelsus: 'All things are toxic; it's the dose that separates the poison from the cure', are the foundation for understanding the dose-response relationship that applies to the occupational health and safety profession.

Important Terms and Concepts

Anaphylaxis - Hypersensitivity resulting from sensitization following prior contact with a chemical or protein.

Antagonistic interaction - Interaction of two chemicals in which the resultant toxic effect is lower than the chemicals' individual actions.

Argyria - A blue-gray discoloration of the skin and deep tissues caused by the deposit of insoluble albuminate of silver. This typically occurs after the medical administration of soluble silver salts over a long period of time.

Atrophy - Stunted development or wasting away of cells and tissue.

Bauxite pneumoconiosis – Known as Shaver's disease. It is caused by inhalation of fumes containing aluminum oxide and silica particles; it is associated with smelting bauxite in the manufacture of corundum.

Biological half-life -The time required to reduce the amount of an externally introduced exogenous substance in the body by half.

Congenital – A health related condition or problem that originates before birth.

Contact dermatitis – Irritation or inflammation of the skin caused by contact with a gaseous, liquid or solid substance. May be caused by primary irritation or an allergy.

Cyanosis – A blue appearance of the skin, most prevalent on the face and extremities, indicating a lack of sufficient oxygen in the arterial blood.

Dose-Response – The correlation between the toxic agent and the effect on the organism.

Enterotoxin - A toxin specific for cells of the intestine that can produce symptoms of food poisoning.

Genetic effects - Mutations or other changes to the germ plasm.

Genetically significant dose (GSD) - The dose that, if received by every member of the population, would be expected to produce the same total genetic injury to the population as the actual doses received by the various individuals.

Hemolysis – The breakdown of red blood cells that result in the liberation of hemoglobin.

LC50 – The lethal concentration. The concentration of a toxic agent in air that kills 50 percent of the test animals within a specified time.

LD50 – The lethal dose. The ingested or injected dose required to produce the death in 50 percent of the exposed population within a specified time.

Liver - The largest gland or organ inside the body. Liver functions include regulating the amino acids in the blood; storing iron and copper for the body; forming and secreting bile; transforming glucose into glycogen; and detoxifying exogenous substances.

Local effect – The reaction due to exposure occurs at the site of exposure.

Malignant – A tumor that is cancerous and capable of undergoing metastasis, which is the invasion of surrounding tissue.

Mitosis – Division of the cell nucleus resulting in nuclei that have the same number and kinds of chromosomes as the original cell.

Mutagen – An agent that can cause a change in the genetic material of a living cell.

Mutation - A transformation of the gene that may result in the alteration of characteristics of offspring.

Peripheral neuropathy – The deterioration of peripheral nerve function that affects the hands, arms, feet, and legs. Certain hydrocarbon solvents cause peripheral neuropathies.

Polycythemia - A condition identified by an excess in the number of red corpuscles in the blood.

Systemic Effect – The reaction due to exposure occurs at a site other than the site of exposure. The reaction site may be called the target organ.

Teratogen – Root meaning 'terrible birth'. An agent or substance that may cause physical defects in the developing embryo or fetus when a pregnant female is exposed to that substance.

Urticaria – Medical term for skin hives.

Zinc protoporphyrin (ZPP) – The hematopoietic enzyme used as a measure of recent lead exposure. Frequently used in combination with blood lead levels to assess employee exposure.

Toxic Agents

Toxic agents can be grouped by exposure route, target organ, or chemical category. The exposure route group categorizes agents by dermal contact, inhalation, and ingestion. Target organ grouping categorizes agents by target toxicity, such as neurotoxic, hepatotoxic, and nephrotoxic. Categorizing toxic agents by chemical category such as metals, pesticides, and organic solvents is based on relatively similar toxic effects occurring in similar substances.

Pesticides

Organophosphates

Greater than 50% of insecticides used are Organophosphorus (OP) compounds, and an assortment of these OPs are among the most extensively used pesticides. OPs can be divided into several subclasses, including phosphates, phosphorothioates, phosphoramidates, and phosphonates.

OP insecticides have high acute toxicity, with oral LD_{50} values in rats below 50 mg/kg. The time interval between exposure and onset of symptoms varies. Muscarinic signs appear first, with nicotinic signs following. Severe OP poisoning normally results in respiratory failure. Mild poisoning and/or early stages of severe poisoning may not show any symptoms. Diagnosis is made through symptom recognition (miosis is observed most often, followed by gastrointestinal symptoms and hypersalivation). The primary target for OPs is acetylcholinesterase (AChE), which is a B-esterase whose physiological role is that of hydrolyzing acetylcholine. It is a major neurotransmitter in the central and peripheral nervous system.

Atropine represents the main treatment for OP poisoning. Atropine is a muscarinic receptor antagonist. It prevents the action of accumulating acetylcholine on these receptors. Oximes [e.g., pralidoxime (2-PAM)] are also used in the therapy of OP poisoning. Treatment for OP dermal exposure is to remove all contaminated clothing and wash the skin with alkaline soap. Several analytical methods are available to measure OPs and their metabolites in body fluids. The parent compound is measured in blood, and metabolites are measured in the urine. *Source: Casarett & Doull's Toxicology The Basic Science of Poisons, 7th Edition*

Carbamates

A variety of carbamate insecticides are derived from carbamic acid. Oral toxicity varies greatly. Carbaryl has low toxicity, and aldicarb has extremely high toxicity. The effects are similar to organophosphates by inhibiting acetylcholinesterase. Skin absorption is low for pure carbamates but becomes an issue due to the solvents and emulsifiers mixed in the various formulations.

Carbamates are not mutagenic or carcinogenic. Fetal toxicity only occurs with maternal toxicity. Most of the formulations have biologically inactive metabolites; however, aldicarb produces sulfoxide and sulfone, which are more potent anticholinesterase agents than aldicarb. The medical treatment for carbamate overexposure is atropine. 2-PAM is not used as it aggravates the toxicity of carbaryl. *Source: Casarett & Doull's Toxicology: The Basic Science of Poisons, 7th Edition*

Organic Solvents

Organic solvents include compounds routinely used in industry. They share the chemical structure of at least one carbon and one hydrogen. Characteristics of organic solvents include a low molecular weight, lipophilicity, and volatility. Solvents dissolve oils, fats, rubber, and plastic.

Solvents are categorized by structure: 1) Aliphatic-carbon chains and 2) Aromatic-ring structure. Short-term, high concentration exposure produces acute health effects by targeting the central nervous system and peripheral nervous system. Long-term, low concentration exposures produce chronic subclinical and clinical effects on the central nervous system, peripheral nervous system, and liver. Some solvents are classified as carcinogens (benzene, carbon tetrachloride), reproductive hazards (methylene chloride), neurotoxins (hexane), and dermatitis. Most organic solvents share the same metabolic pathway, which increases the effects of exposure to mixtures.

Benzene

Health effects include central nervous system depression, hematotoxicity, immunotoxicity, and carcinogenicity. Metabolites (phenol) are the likely cause of toxicity.

Carbon Tetrachloride

Health effects include central nervous system depression and strong liver toxicity. CCl_4 can sensitize the myocardium to catecholamines leading to cardiac arrest. Exposure occurs via inhalation and skin absorption. The metabolites are the likely cause of toxicity. The cytochrome P-450 pathway produces the trichloromethyl free radical, carbon monoxide, chloroform, and phosgene. Acetylcysteine administration can reduce the complications of exposure. The effects are synergistic with ethanol, carbon tetrachloride, isopropyl alcohol, and methanol.

Hexane, n-Hexane

Health effects include low acute toxicity, but chronic exposure can result in peripheral neuropathy that is distal and symmetrical. Metabolites like 2,5-hexanedione contribute to toxic effects. A slow recovery may be possible after removal from exposure.

Methanol

Health effects include central nervous system depression, metabolic acidosis, and ocular toxicity. Metabolic formation of formic acid, formaldehyde, and s-glutathione lead to toxic effects that can be absorbed via inhalation and skin contact. Ethanol can be used as a treatment for acute methanol toxicity as the chemicals compete for target sites with ethanol being biologically preferential (antagonistic effect).

Methylene Chloride

Health effects include eye, skin and respiratory tract irritation, as well as central nervous system depression. It is a potential myocardium sensitizer. Exposure to high concentrations may result in narcosis. Metabolism occurs via two pathways: 1) Cytochrome P-450 metabolites include CO, which leads to increased carboxyhemoglobin, 2) Glutathione metabolites include formic acid and formaldehyde.

Methyl Ethyl Ketone (MEK)

MEK has relatively low acute toxicity. It is not a neurotoxic, carcinogenic or reproductive hazard.

Toluene

Health effects include eye, skin and respiratory tract irritation, as well as central nervous system depression. Chronic high exposures are associated with renal tubule damage.

Metals

Trace metals, heavy metals, and toxic metals are interchangeable terms used to describe a group of metallic elements that can be hazardous if taken into the body. The term *"trace metals"* refers to metals that are present in the environment or in the human body in very low concentrations, such as copper, iron, and zinc. *Heavy metals* are trace metals whose densities are at least five times greater than water, including cadmium, lead, and mercury. *Toxic metals* are metals whose concentrations in the environment are considered harmful.

Specific metals are essential for good health, and their defects can lead to disease. Metals necessary for good health in small amounts can become toxic if ingested in large doses. Metals are unique among pollutant toxicants in that they are all naturally occurring and abundant within the human environment. Other metals have no known functions in the body, and an internal exposure may be harmful. Once metals are in the environment, they find ways into the body through drinking water, food, and inhaled air.

Metals exert their effects in many ways, but usually within body cells. Some metals disrupt chemical reactions, others block the absorption of essential nutrients, and others change the shapes of vital chemical compounds, thus rendering them useless. Some metals bind to nutrients in the stomach and prevent their absorption into the body. Workers exposed to metals on the job may suffer lung damage, skin reactions, and gastrointestinal symptoms from brief contact with high concentrations. Some metals accumulate in the body over time and reach toxic concentrations after years of exposure.

Other human health effects to metals are described below.

Arsenic

Arsenic is a potent carcinogen (lung cancer). Health effects include poisoning via inhalation and ingestion. There is also potential for damage to the peripheral nervous system.

Beryllium

Beryllium exposure may cause the following effects in humans: dermatitis, acute pneumonitis, and chronic pulmonary granulomatosis (berylliosis).

Cadmium

Health effects include kidney disease with chronic exposure and an increased risk of cancer. Exposure to airborne cadmium is associated with nephrotoxicity. In ambient air, cadmium vapor is oxidized rapidly to produce cadmium oxide. Cadmium oxide fumes are a severe pulmonary irritant. Cadmium dust is less of a pulmonary irritant than cadmium oxide fumes because it has a larger particle size.

Chromium

Water soluble hexavalent chromium compounds (e.g., acid mist and chromate dusts) are severe irritants of the nasopharynx, larynx, lungs, and skin. Certain hexavalent compound (e.g., water-insoluble) exposure is directly related to an increased risk of lung cancer.

Lead

Exposure to lead or its inorganic compounds may cause the following effects in humans: severe gastrointestinal disturbances, anemia, neuromuscular dysfunction, and encephalopathy. Lead poisoning symptoms include weakness, weight loss, lassitude, insomnia and hypotension.

Mercury

Inhalation of mercury vapor may produce a metal-fume-fever-like syndrome, including chills, nausea, general malaise, tightness in chest, and respiratory symptoms. High concentrations of the vapor cause corrosive bronchitis and interstitial pneumonitis. In severe cases, subjects can succumb to respiratory insufficiency. Acute exposure to high concentrations of mercury vapor causes severe respiratory damage, whereas chronic exposure to lower levels is associated primarily with central nervous system damage. *Sources: (1) Toxics A-Z; Toxicology, The Basic Science of Poisons. (2) Patty's Toxicology 5th edition, Volume 2. (3) Casarett & Doull's Toxicology, The Basic Science of Poisons, 7th Edition.*

Kinetics
Toxicokinetics is the study of the time course and spatial distribution of a toxin in the body, and includes the following:

- *Absorption*: Movement of the toxin from the site of contact with the body to the blood.
- *Distribution*: Movement of the toxin from the site of absorption to the rest of the body.
- *Metabolism*: Process that occurs within the body (most often the liver) to chemically alter the toxin to a more hydrophilic compound (metabolite).
- *Excretion*: Removal of the toxin or its metabolite from the body, usually in the urine or feces.

A basic assumption is that there is a proportional relationship between the concentration of a substance at the site of toxicity and the concentration of the substance (or metabolite of the substance) as measured in the plasma, urine, or other definable compartment of the body.

Mathematical principles are used to define non-compartmental parameters (algebraic equations) and compartmental models (linear and nonlinear equations) that can predict and describe the concentration of a toxin in the body. The simplest model that predicts accurate changes in concentrations over time should be used.

Non-compartmental parameters include clearance of a toxin from a system (the body), half-life, and volume of distribution.

- No assumption regarding the number of compartments
- Assumes elimination follows first order – the amount removed over a set amount of time is proportional to the total amount in the body

One compartment model: Toxin distributes equally into all tissue and develops a homeostasis throughout.

- The substance distributes completely and instantaneously throughout all tissues in the body – thus the entire body is the one compartment.
- Elimination from the body is first order.

Two or multi-compartment model: A two- compartment model is used to predict tissue toxin concentrations for a substance that distributes quickly into a particular tissue and does not readily redistribute into the plasma or throughout the body.

If distribution and elimination occur in multiple tissues at differing rates, a multi-compartment model is needed.

Example: Substances that are much more soluble in fat will rapidly distribute into adipose tissue but will not redistribute quickly to plasma (water based). Two compartments would need to be used to adequately determine the toxicokinetics: the adipose tissue, and the rest of the body that is predominantly water.

Rubric 16: Toxicology Questions

1. The signs and symptoms of acute organophosphate poisoning include:

    A) Nausea, drowsiness, irritation of the mucous membrane, and dilation of the pupils.
    B) Nausea, abdominal cramps, increased salivation, increased lacrimation, and broncho-constriction.
    C) Euphoria, dizziness, pain and swelling of the joints.
    D) Lethargy, cyanosis, bronchodilation, and gastrointestinal bleeding.

2. Which of the following can cause damage to the bone marrow following prolonged exposure?

    A) Carbon dioxide.
    B) Lead.
    C) Toluene Diisocyanate.
    D) Beryllium.

3. A teratogen is best described by the following statement:

    A) An agent that causes a genetic mutation.
    B) An agent that increases cellular proliferation.
    C) An agent that causes congenital malformation.
    D) A chemical that causes cancer.

4. Which of the following particles of SiO2 would be most harmful if inhaled?

    A) Those with a diameter of 2 to 5um.
    B) Those with a diameter of 0.5 um.
    C) Those with a diameter above 10 um.
    D) Those with a diameter below 0.5 um.

5. Which of the following is not used as biological exposure index, (BEI), in a biological monitoring program?

    A) Blood.
    B) Exhaled air.
    C) Lymphatic tissue.
    D) Urine.

6. Which layer of the epidermis is most important in dermal absorption?

    A) Stratum spinosum.
    B) Stratum corneum.
    C) Basal layer.
    D) Multipilagian layer.

7. A 50-year-old sculptor is complaining of shortness of breath. His chest x-ray reveals fibrotic changes in the upper lobes of his lungs. These lungs are most likely associated with:

    A) Asbestos exposure.
    B) Silica exposure.
    C) Aluminum exposure.
    D) Organic vapor exposure.

8. What effect does water solubility have on the site of action for inhaled chemicals?

    A) Less solubility/less penetration into lungs.
    B) Greater solubility/greater penetration into lungs.
    C) Greater solubility/less penetration into lungs.
    D) Solubility does not affect penetration.

9. Which of the following is not associated with decreased sperm count in humans?

    A) Ethylene dibromide.
    B) Dibromochloropropane.
    C) Formaldehyde.
    D) Lead.

10. Formaldehyde is best described as a:

    A) Secondary irritant.
    B) CNS depressant.
    C) Primary irritant.
    D) CNS stimulant.

11. Which of the following is not true about benzene?

    A) Quinone is a metabolite.
    B) Can cause aplastic anemia.
    C) Rapidly absorbed through the skin.
    D) Excreted in urine as phenol.

12. Which of the following is typical of methemoglobinemia?

    A) Heme iron is oxidized from ferrous to ferril state.
    B) Heme iron is oxidized from ferril to ferrous state.
    C) Heme iron is reduced from ferril to ferrous.
    D) Occurs only in vitro.

13. When evaluating the dose response curve for 2 substances, with dose on the x-axis and response on the y-axis, substance A has a steeper LD_{50} slope than substance B. This indicates:

    A) Substance A is less toxic than substance B.
    B) Substance A has no minimum safe dose.
    C) Substance B is non-toxic.
    D) Substance A is more toxic than substance B.

14. The recommended biological monitoring technique for evaluating styrene is:

    A) Total phenol in urine.
    B) Mandelic acid in urine.
    C) Mandelic acid in blood.
    D) Hippicuric acid in urine.

15. Occupational cadmium poisoning is best described by the following statement:

    A) Headache, dizziness, nausea, blurred vision, tachycardia, and bright red coloration of the mucous membrane.
    B) Headache, vertigo, weakness, cyanosis, tremor, and brownish urine.
    C) Anorexia, constipation, irritability, abdominal tenderness, and elevated protoporphyrin.
    D) Cough, chest pain, dyspnea, and pulmonary edema.

16. What effect would be expected following hydration of the stratum corneum?

    A) Decreases in permeability.
    B) It becomes harder.
    C) Destratification.
    D) It increases permeability approximately 10 fold.

17. Generally, it takes _____ half-lives to eliminate a toxin from the body.

    A) 1
    B) 5-10
    C) 100-200
    D) 1000-10,000

18. A compound is more likely to move via passive transport across cell membranes if:

    A) Lipid soluble.
    B) Lipid insoluble.
    C) High pH.
    D) Low pH.

19. An autopsy of a male who worked in the electroplating industry for 30 years revealed significant kidney damage. Cadmium exposure is likely. Which specific area of the kidney should be damaged?

    A) Distal renal tubules.
    B) Ureter.
    C) Proximal renal tubules.
    D) Efferent arteriole.

20. The painful joint and spine condition known as itai-itai was identified in 1912 in Japan. The cause was identified later as:

    A) Lead poisoning.
    B) Keto-acidosis.
    C) Cadmium poisoning.
    D) Cold and damp conditions.

Rubric 16: Toxicology Answers

1. Answer: B
Explanation: Inhibition of acetylcholinesterase results in broncho-constriction, wheezing, increased salivation, increased lacrimation, nausea, vomiting, abdominal cramps, diarrhea, and bradycardia, but DOES NOT CAUSE swelling, bronchodilation, irritation of mucous membranes, or dilation of pupils.

2. Answer: B
Explanation: Overexposure to lead may damage the bone marrow. Carbon dioxide is relatively non-toxic, TDI is a sensitizer, and beryllium exposure may result in lung disease.

3. Answer: C
Explanation: Mutagens cause genetic mutations. Teratogen is the production of abnormal offspring.

4. Answer: A
Explanation: Particles with a diameter of 2 – 5 microns are deposited in the alveolar region. Particles less than 0.5 microns are also deposited, but their overall mass is so small that the health impact is minimal. Particles with a 10-micron diameter tend to be filtered in the upper respiratory system.

5. Answer: C
Explanation: To be acceptable, BEI samples must be minimally invasive. A biopsy of lymph tissue is invasive.

6. Answer: B
Explanation: The stratum corneum is the outer layer of keratinized cells in a lipid matrix.

7. Answer: B
Explanation: A sculptor is more likely to have silica exposure than asbestos. The chest x-rays are consistent with silicosis.

8. Answer C
Explanation: More soluble substances react with water in upper airway, throat, etc. However, they do not penetrate as deeply.

9. Answer: C
Explanation: All but formaldehyde are associated with decreased sperm count.

10. Answer: C
Explanation: Formaldehyde is very soluble in water, thus increasing its irritant ability.

11. Answer: C

Explanation: Benzene is metabolized to quinone and semiquinone via the P-450 pathway before being excreted in exhaled air or in urine as phenol.

12. Answer: A

Explanation: Chemical oxidation involving a valence change from ferrous to ferric state creates the brownish-black pigment, methemoglobin.

13. Answer: D

Explanation: The dose response curve is a classic toxicology tool. Steeper slope indicates a more rapid toxic effect.

14. Answer: B

Explanation: The ACGIH recommends mandelic acid in urine.

15. Answer: D

Explanation: Answer A is CO poisoning and answer C is lead poisoning. Answer B is a mixture of symptoms.

16. Answer: D

Explanation: Hydration increases permeability, which increases risk of overexposure in hot/humid or wet work environments.

17. Answer: B

Explanation: A blood concentration of x= 100 ug/Dl will be 0.75 ug/Dl after 7 half-lives.

18. Answer: A

Explanation: The rate of transfer is dependent on the lipid-water partition coefficient. The pH-partition theory states that lipid-soluble, non-ionized compounds will transport passively.

19. Answer: C

Explanation: Tubular degeneration is the most common morphological finding, especially in the proximal tubules.

20. Answer: C

Explanation: Itai-itai, known as it-hurts or ouch-ouch, was caused by cadmium in mine runoff. The water from the Jinzu River was used for irrigation of rice. The rice absorbed metals such as cadmium, which lead to prolonged ingestion of cadmium and the weakening of the bones. *Sources: (1)Patty's Toxicology Vol 1,2,3. 5th ed. (2) Casarett and Doull's Toxicology 7th ed.*

Rubric 17: Work Environments and Industrial Processes

The occupational hygienist must be able to apply skills and knowledge to many industrial and occupational environments. Some of the environments are classical industrial settings while some are recent developments.

Foundry

Foundries are manufacturing processes that cast metal into shapes by melting to a liquid, pouring in a mold, and removing the mold from the cast object. The most common metals processed are aluminum and cast iron. Other metals used to produce castings in foundries include bronze, steel, magnesium, copper, tin, and zinc. The metal casting process is broken down into five categories: mold preparation; metal preparation and pouring; transfer, pouring, cooling; shakeout - the separation of the solid- but still not cold- casting from its molding sand; and cleaning and finishing.

The metal casting process has the potential to expose workers to a variety of hazards in foundries. Hazards include exposures to dust; metal fumes; carbon monoxide; resin bonding chemicals; noise; vibration; heat; and coke. Coke is a solid carbonaceous material derived from destructive distillation of low-ash, low-sulfur bituminous coal. Coke is used as a fuel and as a reducing agent on smelting iron ore in a blast furnace. It is there to reduce the iron oxide (hematite) to collect iron.

Metalworking

Metalworking is the process of working with metals to create individual parts, assemblies, or large structures. Machining metalworking involves milling metals. Milling is the shaping of metal or other materials by eliminating material to form the final shape. This process is normally done on a milling machine.

Metalworking fluids (MWFs) reduce heat and friction, and remove metal particles in industrial machining and grinding operations. MWFs may be mixtures of oils, emulsifiers, anti-weld agents, corrosion inhibitors, pressure additives, buffers, biocides and other components. Workers in machine finishing, machine tooling, and other metal-forming operations are potentially exposed. Adverse health effects can occur following skin contact with contaminated materials, spray, or mist, and by breathing MWF mist or aerosol. Skin irritation, dermatitis, acne, lung irritation, asthma, hypersensitivity pneumonitis, and possibly cancer health problems are associated with skin and airborne exposures to MWFs.

Pulp-Paper Manufacture

The manufacture of pulp and paper is one of the world's oldest and largest industries. The basic pulp-paper manufacturing is a process that transforms wood chips into pulp. Two types of pulping are chemical and mechanical pulping. Chemical pulping is the breakdown of the chemical structure of lignin so the lignin may be washed from the cellulose fibers. Lignin holds the plant cells together, but chemical pulping frees the fibers and makes pulp. Mechanical pulping involves two types of mechanical pulps: thermo-mechanical pulp (TMP) and groundwood pulp processes. A thermo-mechanical pulp processes chipped wood that is fed into large steam-heated refiners where the chips are squeezed and turned into fibers. In groundwood processes, debarked logs are fed into grinders where they are pressed against rotating stones and reduced into fibers.

Workers can be exposed to a variety of hazards in pulp-paper manufacturing. During the Kraft process, the digester is opened and contents are dumped, thus creating potential exposures to hydrogen sulfide, methyl mercaptan, dimethyl sulfide, dimethyl disulfide, and sulfur dioxide. Potential exposure to chlorine and chlorine dioxide is possible during bleaching operations.

Plastic

Plastics are materials that utilize an organic substance of large molecular weight as a substrate. Two industrial plastic processes are *thermosetting*, which is irreversibly rigid, and *thermoplastic*, which is reversibly rigid. Plastics are called resins or synthetic resins prior to compounding and processing. Examples of plastics include vinyl, acrylic, polyethylene, phenolics, ureas, and melamine. Plastic processing is performed by three methods: compression molding, injection molding, and extrusion.

The hazards associated with plastic production include routine temperatures of 390-570 degrees Fahrenheit. If higher temperatures are encountered, then thermal degradation products will be released. Hydrogen chloride is released from polyvinyl chloride, styrene from polystyrene, nitrogen containing compounds from nylon and acrylonitrile, fluoride compounds from PTFE (polytetrafluoroethylene), and cyanide compounds from urethanes. Physical hazards may include heat and noise. Plastic particles can create combustible dust hazards.

Ceramic

The term ceramic identifies an inorganic, non-metallic solid prepared by the action of heat and subsequent cooling, which is applied to pottery, brick, and tile products molded from clay and then calcined. Ceramic materials may have a crystalline or partly crystalline structure, or amorphous (e.g., a glass). Ceramics are produced from clay and other minerals, and are fired in a kiln to give permanence of shape and mechanical strength. Potential exposure to ceramic production includes inhalation of respirable dust, heat, radiation, and toxic emissions from kilns.

Glass is a ceramic product. Glass or silica sand (washed) has the potential to cause silicosis. Silicosis is uncommon in modern-day plants, but there can be a dust hazard due to bulk handling. Refractory ceramic fiber is high temperature insulation wool. Ceramic fiber is manufactured from aluminum silicate glass used for thermal insulation in high temperature applications and processes up to 700°C.

Degreasing

Degreasing is the removal of surface grime, oil, and grease from metal and plastic with solvents and cleaners. The table below describes the route of entry and hazard associated with degreasing and vapor degreasers.

Processes and Hazards by Route of Entry

Unit Process	Route of Entry and Hazard
Degreasing - Removing grease, oil, and dirt from metal and plastic with solvents and cleaners. **Cold solvent washing** - Clean parts with ketones, cellosolves, aliphatic, aromatic, and stoddard solvents.	**Inhalation** – Vapors. **Skin contact** - Dermatitis and absorption. **Fire and explosion (if flammable).** **Metabolic** - Carbon monoxide formed with methylene chloride.
Vapor degreasers - Trichloroethylene, methyl chloroform, ethylene dichloride, and certain fluorocarbon compounds.	**Inhalation** – (1) Vapors; (2) Thermal degradation may form phosgene, hydrogen chloride, and chlorine gases. **Skin contact** - Dermatitis and absorption.

Vapor degreasing involves heating a solvent to its boiling point. The solvent vapor rises and fills the tank to an elevation determined by the location of a condenser. Finally, the vapor condenses and returns to the liquid sump.

Abrasive Blasting

Abrasive blasting is a process for cleaning surfaces with sand, alumina, or steel grit in a stream of high-pressure air. Abrasive blasting is a significant source of metal exposure. Abrasive blasting is categorized into three groups: air, hydroblast, and centrifugal impeller. Multiple substances can be used for abrasive blasting. The substances include metallurgical slags (copper, nickel, zinc), metal grit (iron and steel), aluminum oxide, plastic beads, sodium bicarbonate, metal shot (bronze, steel, stainless steel), garnet, organic materials, sand, and dry ice. Health hazards of abrasive blasting include silicosis (silica sand), metals (slag and heavy metals), and hazards due to substrate removal (Pb, Cr).

Petroleum-Chemical Refining

Refining is the processing of one complex mixture of hydrocarbon into a number of other complex mixtures of hydrocarbons. The crude oil is processed into flammable gases and liquids at high temperatures and pressures using vessels, equipment, and piping. Refineries produce a variety of products, including many required as a raw material product for the petrochemical industry.

There are four main processes associated with refinery work. The hazards associated with each process are described below.

The distillation process produces kerosene by simple atmospheric distillation. Hazards associated with this process include aromatic hydrocarbons, hydrogen sulfide (H_2S), and noise.

The thermal cracking process exposes heavy fuels to pressure and intense heat, which physically breaks down the large molecules into smaller ones to produce gasoline and distillate fuels. Hazards associated with this process include benzene, naphtha, carbon monoxide (CO), noise, and catalysts.

The catalytic and polymerization processes make it possible to provide improved gasoline yields and higher octane numbers for the higher-compression gasoline engines. Hazards associated with this process include hydrogen fluoride (HF), sulfuric acid, naphthas, noise, and acid sludge.

The isomerization process converts linear molecules to higher-octane branch molecules for blending into gasoline or feeding to alkylation units. Hazards associated with this process include benzene and light naphthas.

Hydrocarbon chemistry is complex, and the risk of fire and explosion is a major concern in the petrochemical and refining industries.

Tanning

Tanning is a process of taking an animal hide to a usable leather. This process encompasses four distinct steps, including drying, soaking pits, beam-house operations, and tanning. The steps are described below.
- **Drying**: Flints- dried hides, curing dry-salting (saturated sodium chloride).
- **Soaking pits** (to loosen up dried hides): Caustic soda disinfectants.
- **"Beam-house" operations**: Liming (loosen epidermis, hair roots, proteins, fats).
- **Fleshing/removing hair**.
- **De-liming or bathing** (weak acid or ammonium solution).
- **Tanning**: Converts hides to usable leather by stabilization.
  - Two methods: Vegetable (Tannin) and Chrome.

Potential exposure to various hazards when working in tanneries include acids (acetic, chromic, formic, hydrochloric, oxalic, phenol, and sulfuric), ammonia, caustics (soda ash, sodium hydroxide, sodium sulfide), and contact dermatitis from raw hides.

Textile

Textiles are either natural or synthetic. They can be woven fabrics, knit or terry cloth, and may be coated with rubber or plastic.

Cotton dust is a hazard to workers in the textile industry. Cotton dust exposure can result in Byssinosis, which is an acute chest tightness that recurs at the beginning of each workweek, lasts 1-2 days in the early stages, and eventually becomes a chronic, disabling respiratory disease. Cotton may also be contaminated with gram-negative bacteria endotoxins that cause acute respiratory symptoms and pulmonary function decline.

The following describes the process of how to produce cotton:

- **Opening**: Preliminary treatment of raw cotton, Separation of compressed and matted masses into loose tufts and removal of heavier and bulkier impurities.
- **Picking**: Further opening and cleaning of stock and formation of a continuous mat (called a lap).
- **Carding**: Removing most of the impurities and some of the short, broken or immature fibers and arrangement into a thin lacy web and then into a thin light sliver.
- **Drawing**: Improvement of the uniformity of the silver and arrangement of fibers into parallel order.
- **Combing**: Removal of short fibers.
- **Roving**.
- **Spinning**.

Welding

Welding involves melting of a metal by either a flame or electric arc in the presence of a flux or shielding gas. The types of welding include electric arc-welding, oxyacetylene welding, spot welding, and inert or shielded gas welding using helium or argon. The hazards involved in welding stem from the fumes from the weld metal, such as lead or cadmium metal, the gases created by the process, and the fumes or gases arising from the flux.

Electroplating/Anodizing

Electroplating and anodizing entail metal, plastic and rubber parts that are plated to prevent rusting and corrosion, to reduce electrical contact resistance, to provide electrical insulation, and to improve durability.

Anodizing is utilized for surface treatment as decoration, corrosion resistance, and electrical insulation on metals (magnesium, aluminum and titanium).

Electroplating is a chemical or electrochemical process wherein a metallic layer is deposited on the surface of a base material.

Battery (Lead Acid) Manufacturing

Battery manufacturing includes the making of rechargeable or accumulator batteries that consist of a series of identical cells that each deliver the same voltage (1.5-2 volts/cell). Cells entail positive and negative plates in an electrolyte. Exposures in the battery manufacturer process include exposure to lead and lead compounds during paste mixing and pasting. Lead may be melted and cast creating exposures to heat and lead fumes. The electrolyte is usually sulfuric acid. Hazards potentially produced include exposure to arsenic (contaminant) and arsine, and hydrogen gas during battery charging.

Indoor Air Quality (IAQ)

Three most common IAQ contaminants are volatile or reactive chemicals, pollen, microbial agents, or bio-organic toxins. Remedial methods include increasing air mixing, adding more outside air, rearranging building occupancy, and reconfiguring air handling equipment. Potential exposures associated with IAQ issues include ozone, NO_2, CO_2, CO, organic chemicals, fibers, and SO_2.

Rubric 17: Work Environments and Industrial Processes Questions

1. Foundries are classical heavy industries in which metals are cast into shapes by melting into a liquid, pouring into a mold, and removing the mold from the cast object. Historically, ferrous foundries have utilized sand for creating molds. Select the most common hazard outcomes found in this type of foundry.

    A) Ionizing radiation and metal fume exposure resulting in erythema and an acute flu-like illness.
    B) Iron oxide and silica exposure resulting in siderosis and silicosis.
    C) Lead oxide and coal dust exposure resulting in bone marrow disease and pneumoconiosis.
    D) Heat and solvent exposure resulting in heat stress and cirrhosis of the liver.

2. Coal dust is sometimes found in the mold sand. This results in the generation of _____ during the cooling of the metal casting.

    A) Airborne coal dust.
    B) Carbon monoxide.
    C) Bitumen fume.
    D) Coal oil gas.

3. Three foundry workers arrive at the nurse's office complaining of headaches, nausea, and dizziness. Their breathing appears rapid. Select the likely cause of the symptoms.

    A) Inhalation of formaldehyde and furfuryl alcohol.
    B) Inhalation of carbon monoxide.
    C) Inhalation of metal fumes.
    D) Food poisoning.

4. Metal working fluids are used to reduce heat and friction, thereby improving product quality in the machining process. There are several formulations of metal working fluids, one of which is called straight oil. Straight oil is best described as:

    A) Synthetic fluid.
    B) Petroleum fluid.
    C) Water based fluid.
    D) Semi-synthetic fluid.

5. Pulp-paper manufacturing may utilize the Kraft process. The Kraft process utilizes a mixture of sodium hydroxide and sodium sulfide (white liquor) that breaks links between lignin and cellulose. Exposures occur when workers open the bottom of the digester and dump the contents. What exposures can be anticipated during this activity?

    A) Hydrogen chloride, calcium chloride.
    B) Hydrogen sulfide, sulfur dioxide.
    C) Hydrogen cyanide, sodium cyanide.
    D) Hydrogen, chlorine.

6. Excess moisture in buildings is problematic. In addition to condensation stains and clogging salt shakers, warm/humid environments allow mold to thrive. In warm/humid environments, moisture originates in the structure but primarily enters from outside by infiltration and ventilation. Once inside, condensation can occur. Select the best techniques to control the indoor humidity and reduce condensation in this climate.

   A) Install insulation in the wall cavity with a vapor barrier on the outer (warm side) of the wall.
   B) Install insulation in the wall cavity with a vapor barrier on the inner (cool side) of the wall.
   C) Install a dehumidifier in the crawlspace of the building.
   D) Install the insulation in the wall cavity and utilize rubberized or impermeable wall coverings on the inner (cool side) of the wall.

7. Gas Tungsten Metal Arc Welding (GTAW) is the preferred term for TIG welding. It involves the coalescence of metals by heating with an arc between the tungsten rod and the work. Shielding is provided by a gas or gas mixture. The tungsten rod may contain several percent of the following:

   A) Beryllium.
   B) Thorium.
   C) Polonium.
   D) Ruthenium.

8. Natural gas and liquefied petroleum gas are colorless and have no odor. To improve detection of the presence of these flammable gases, an odorizing agent is added. Select the common odorizing agent.

   A) Ethyl mercaptan.
   B) Sulfur dioxide.
   C) Hydrogen sulfide.
   D) Sulfur trioxide.

9. Which of the following would not be produced by plasma arc welding?

   A) Ozone.
   B) UV light.
   C) Infrared radiation.
   D) Metal dusts.

10. ASHRAE 62-2010 is primarily a design standard that specifies 7-20 cfm outdoor air per person by occupancy. It also lists a target level for carbon dioxide. Why is a carbon dioxide level specified?

   A) It is highly toxic.
   B) It is exhaled by occupants and is a chemical asphyxiant.
   C) The level of carbon dioxide may parallel the level of other contaminants.
   D) It indicates the presence of biological contamination.

11. Cotton textile workers are at risk for developing the following disease:

    A) Halitosis.
    B) Black lung.
    C) Mesothelioma.
    D) Byssinosis.

12. The person designated by the employer to provide technical guidance of the Chemical Hygiene Plan holds what title?

    A) Industrial Hygiene Officer.
    B) Chemical Hygiene Officer.
    C) Chemical Safety Officer.
    D) Environmental Health Manager.

13. Which of the following agents should not contribute to indoor air pollution?

    A) Carbon dioxide.
    B) Formaldehyde.
    C) Asbestos.
    D) PCBs.

14. An office building serves 100 occupants. The building HVAC system supplies 10,000 CFM. What is the outdoor air ventilation rate per person if the building HVAC system supplies 10,000 CFM, and 80% of the air is recirculated?

    A) 0 CFM/person.
    B) 10 CFM/person.
    C) 20 CFM/person.
    D) 30 CFM/person.

15. Chromium and chromium compounds are usually not found in which of the following industries or occupations?

    A) Metal plating.
    B) Welding processes.
    C) Stainless steel production and use.
    D) Agriculture processes.

16. Choose the answer that provides the best control measure for reducing dermatitis in electroplaters.

    A) Gloves.
    B) Local exhaust ventilation.
    C) Frequent hand washing.
    D) Barrier creams.

17. Solvents in the form of a(n) _____ is useful for degreasing chemicals.

    A) Vapor.
    B) Liquid.
    C) Gas.
    D) Aerosol.

18. An employee of a battery recycling company had the task of recycling car batteries' melted slag. The employee did not deem it necessary to wear appropriate personal protective equipment while performing the task, and the company did not monitor the situation. Choose the primary risk for this task.

    A) Lead poisoning.
    B) Burns and abrasions on skin.
    C) Burns caused by infrared or intense radiant light.
    D) Iron poisoning.

19. Which of the following answer choices is a good indicator for determining the adequacy of outdoor air exchange in buildings?

    A) Carbon dioxide.
    B) Nitrogen.
    C) Carbon monoxide.
    D) Oxygen.

20. A worker applying polyurethane paint in a paint booth has been complaining of eye, nose, throat irritation, and chest pain. What is the likely cause of the worker's complications?

    A) Toluene diisocyanate exposure.
    B) Methyl chloride exposure.
    C) Cyclohexane exposure.
    D) Boron oxide exposure.

1. Answer: B
Explanation: Some studies suggest that ferrous (iron) foundries that use sand molds are the leading industry for silicosis cases. Siderosis is a condition of iron accumulation in the lungs that becomes visible on x-ray and is associated with the inhalation of iron oxide fumes. Metal fume fever is present in ferrous foundries but not to the extent of silicosis and siderosis. Ionizing radiation is not a significant exposure in foundries. *Source: Foundry Health Hazards publication, NOHSC, Government of Australia*

2. Answer: B
Explanation: The heat of the cast metal combusts the coal dust, thus producing carbon monoxide. *Source: Foundry Health Hazards publication, NOHSC, Government of Australia*

3. Answer: B
Explanation: In addition to the above symptoms, carbon monoxide exposure can lead to mental confusion and increase the risk of other injuries and accidents. *Source: Foundry Health Hazards publication, NOHSC, Government of Australia*

4. Answer: B
Explanation: There are four major classes of metal-working fluids widely available: straight oil, soluble oil, semisynthetic, and synthetic. Many metalworking fluids, except the straight oils, are mixed with water for use. Each has additives such as surfactants, biocides, extreme pressure agents, anti-oxidants, and corrosion inhibitors to improve performance and increase fluid life (refer to Appendix 2 for a listing of typical additives).

Straight Oil: This type of metalworking fluid is comprised mostly of mineral (petroleum) or vegetable oils. Petroleum oils used for these fluids today tend to be "severely solvent refined" or "severely hydrotreated" (refining processes that reduce cancer-causing substances called polynuclear aromatic hydrocarbons [PAHs] present in crude oil). Other oils of animal, marine or synthetic origin can also be used singularly or in combination with straight oils to increase the wetting action and lubricity. Straight oils can be recognized by an oily appearance and viscous feel. These materials may contain chlorinated and sulfur additives. This product is not diluted with water before use. Straight-oil metalworking fluids are generally used for processes that require lubrication rather than cooling. They perform best when used at slow cut speeds, high metal-to-metal contact, or with older machines made specifically for use with straight oils. Straight-oil MWF systems may require fire protection.

Soluble Oil: Soluble oil is also called emulsifiable oil. It is comprised of 30 to 85 percent of severely refined lubricant base oil and emulsifiers to help disperse the oil in water. The fluid concentrate usually includes other additives to improve performance and lengthen the life of the fluid. Soluble oil products are supplied as concentrates that are diluted with water to obtain the working fluid. They may have colorants added. Soluble oils provide good lubrication and are better at cooling than straight oils. Drawbacks in using soluble oils include poor corrosion control, are sometimes "dirty" (i.e., machine tool surfaces and nearby areas become covered with oil or difficult-to-remove product residues), may smoke (they may not cool as well as semisynthetics and synthetics), and may have poor mix stability or short sump life.

Semi-synthetic: This type of metalworking fluid contains a lower amount of severely refined base oil, such as 5-30 percent in the concentrate. Semi-synthetics offer good lubrication, good heat reduction, good rust control, have longer sump life, and are cleaner than soluble oils. They have many of the same ingredients as soluble oils and contain a more complex emulsifier package.

Synthetic: These metalworking fluid formulations do not contain any petroleum oil. They contain detergent-like components to help "wet" the part and other additives to improve performance. Like the other classes of water-miscible fluids, synthetics are designed to be diluted with water. *Source: OSHA Metal Working Fluid Manual*

5. Answer: B
Explanation: This task has potential exposure to hydrogen sulfide, methyl mercaptan, dimethyl sulfide, dimethyl disulfide, and sulfur dioxide. Bleaching operations produce chlorine and chlorine dioxide. *Source: Forest Products Chemistry. Papermaking Science and Technology*

6. Answer: A
Explanation: In warm, humid climates preventing the moist outside air from migrating into the wall cavity is important. By placing the vapor barrier on the outside of the wall, moisture and condensation within the wall is reduced.

A vapor barrier on the inside wall promotes condensation within the wall when warm, humid air contacts the vapor barrier that is cooled by indoor air conditioning.

A crawlspace dehumidifier will reduce moisture under the structure but is not a common approach. It does not control infiltration; rather, it reduces moisture from a defined area.

Impermeable interior wall coverings in this climate promote condensation within the wall when warm, humid air contacts the vapor barrier that is cooled by indoor air conditioning.

Ventilation should be used in bathrooms, shower rooms, etc., to exhaust humid air. The cooling coils of the HVAC system will remove moisture from the conditioned air. *Source: Clemson University, Moisture: Build to Keep it Out*

7. Answer: B
Explanation: Thorium is a radioactive additive used because the treated rods make high quality, long lasting welds. It is possible, but not common, for a welder to exceed the annual radiation dose based on heavy welding and grinding on this type of weld. Tungsten is not consumed, and fume generation with this type of welding is relatively low. *Source: American Welding Society – Tech Fact 27*

8.   Answer: A
Explanation: Sulfur-containing odorants include:
<u>tert-Butyl thiol (TBM)</u>, the main ingredient in many gas odorant blends.
<u>Tetrahydrothiophene (THT)</u>, used as an odorant for natural gas, usually in mixtures containing tert-butyl thiol.
<u>2-Propanethiol</u>, commonly known as isopropyl mercaptan (IPM) is used as an odorant for natural gas usually in mixtures containing tert-butyl thiol.
<u>Ethanethiol (EM)</u>, commonly known as ethyl mercaptan is used in liquefied petroleum gas (LPG), and resembles odor of leeks, onions, durian, or cooked cabbage.
<u>Dimethyl sulfide (DMS)</u>, a component of the smell produced from cooking of certain vegetables, notably maize, cabbage, beetroot, and seafoods. *Pacific Natural Gas and Odorant Additive information*

9.   Answer: D
Explanation: The metal would be generated as a fume, not a dust. *Source: Patty's Toxicology, Vol 3, 5th edition*

10. Answer: C
Explanation: Carbon dioxide is exhaled by occupants, and as the level of carbon dioxide increases, the level of more harmful contaminants may increase. It is used as an easily detectable indicator of air quality. Levels exceeding 900 ppm have been linked to increased complaints in some studies.

11. Answer: D
Explanation: Byssinosis is an acute chest tightness that occurs at the beginning of each workweek and lasts a few days initially, but can become a chronic debilitating disease over time. The causative agent has been identified as finely pulverized cotton bract (not cotton fiber). It is also called Brown Lung and Monday fever.
                          Source: American Lung Association and University of Utah

12. Answer: B
Explanation: A Chemical Hygiene Officer is an employee designated by the employer, and who is qualified by training or experience, to provide technical guidance in the development and implementation of the provisions of the Chemical Hygiene Plan. *Source: OSHA 29 CFR 1910.1450*

13. Answer: D
Explanation: PCBs have a very low vapor pressure and should not cause indoor air quality complications unless burned. The other agents listed (carbon dioxide, formaldehyde, and asbestos are common indoor air pollutants. *Source: The Occupational Environment: Its Evaluation, Control, and Management, 3rd Edition*

14. Answer: C

Explanation:

Step 1: Determine the amount of outdoor air

$$10,000 \ CFM \ x \ 0.2 = 2,000 \ CFM$$

Step 2: Determine the CFM per person

$$CFM \ per \ person = \frac{2,000 \ CFM}{100 \ people}$$
$$CFM \ per \ person = 20$$

Source: None

15. Answer: D

Agent	Health Effects	Common Industries
Chromium and compounds	- Chromium in the hexavalent oxidation state is the most toxic. - Exposure may be to dust in some operations and mist in electroplating. - Exposure to chromium hexavalent compounds may cause irritation effects, allergic sensitization, and lung cancer.	- Metal plating - Chemical research - Welding - Stainless steel production and use - Machining

16. Answer: A

Explanation: The best control measure for protecting from dermatitis is to prevent contact with agent. Gloves are the best control measure.

17. Answer: A

Explanation: The vapor of a solvent is utilized in the degreasing chemical for removing oils and other contaminants from metals. The vapor is compressed back into a liquid that falls back into a sump where it is heated into a vapor again. *Source: None provided*

18. Answer: A

Explanation: Lead is a lustrous, silvery metal that tarnishes in the presence of air and becomes a dull bluish gray. Uses of lead include storage batteries; paint; ink; ceramics; automobile radiator repair; and ammunition (explosive or firing range). Prolonged absorption of lead or its inorganic compounds results in severe gastrointestinal disturbances and anemia. Neuromuscular dysfunction occurs with more serious intoxication; the most severe lead exposure may result in encephalopathy. *Source: Proctor and Hughes' Chemical Hazards of the Workplace, 3rd Edition*

19. Answer: A

Explanation: If outdoor air make-up and exhaust are balanced, and the zones served by each air handler are separated and well defined, it is possible to estimate the minimum flow of outdoor air to each space and compare it to ventilation standards such as ASHRAE 62-1989. Techniques used for this evaluation include the direct measurement of the outdoor air intake and the calculation of the percentage of outdoor air by a temperature or CO_2 balance. Carbon dioxide measured in an occupied space is also an indicator of ventilation adequacy.

CO_2 is frequently measured to assess the adequacy of ventilation, or as a means of controlling ventilation to auditoriums or other spaces with variable occupancy. *Sources: CDC/NIOSH Appendix B: HVAC Systems and Indoor Air Quality & The Occupational Environment: Its Evaluation, Control, and Management, 3rd Edition*

20. Answer: A

Explanation: Toluene diisocyanate is a colorless liquid in the form of an aerosol. Toluene diisocyanate is used in the production of polyurethane foams and plastics and in polyurethane paints and wire coatings. Toluene diisocyanate (TDI) is a strong irritant of the eyes, mucus membranes and skin. It is a potent sensitizer of the respiratory tract. Other complications include choking sensation cough and chest pain. *Source: Proctor and Hughes' Chemical Hazards of the Workplace, 3rd Edition*

Self-Assessment Exam 1

1. An IH trained in phase contrast microscopy has analyzed a filter for asbestos fiber density on the filter. The calculated fiber density is $381 f/mm^2$. The sample for asbestos was collected over 450 minutes of an 8-hour shift at 2 L/m. Calculate the airborne concentration.

   A) 147 f/mL or 147 f/cc
   B) 0.33 f/mL or 0.33 f/cc
   C) 1 f/mL or 1 f/cc
   D) 0.16 f/mL or 0.16 f/cc

2. Using the lead extended work-shift formula: PEL ($\mu g/m^3$) = 400/hours worked in the day, what is the adjusted PEL for a 10-hour shift?

   A) 45 $\mu g/m^3$
   B) 42 $\mu g/m^3$
   C) 40 $\mu g/m^3$
   D) 33 $\mu g/m^3$

3. Select the most commonly used detector cell for measuring oxygen:

   A) Galvanic.
   B) Metal oxide semiconductor.
   C) Conductivity.
   D) Coulometric.

4. The partial pressures of a mixture of gasses are 66% N_2, 10% O_2, and 24% CO_2 by volume at 1 atmosphere. What is the partial pressure of each gas in mmHg?

   A) N_2 = 501.6 mmHg, O_2 = 76 mmHg, and CO_2 = 182.4 mmHg
   B) N_2 = 0.66 mmHg, O_2 = 0.1 mmHg, and CO_2 = 0.24 mmHg
   C) N_2 = 218 mmHg, O_2 = 218 mmHg, and CO_2 = 324 mmHg
   D) N_2 = 253.3.6 mmHg, O_2 = 253.3 mmHg, and CO_2 = 1253.3 mmHg

5. What is the appropriate method when sampling for Vinyl Chloride?

   A) NIOSH 1007.
   B) NIOSH 1200.
   C) NIOSH 1300.
   D) NIOSH 1301.

6. Select the compound that is least likely to be quantitatively analyzed by infrared spectrophotometry.

    A) Benzo(a)pyrene on an XAD-2 tube.
    B) Oil mist on a PVC filter.
    C) Nitrous oxide in a bag.
    D) Quartz (silica) on a PVC filter.

7. What eye defect develops when the human lens loses its elasticity?

    A) Astigmatism.
    B) Farsightedness.
    C) Presbyopia.
    D) Nearsightedness.

8. The Mars lander is performing chemistry experiments while on the red planet. Calculate the molar volume under the following conditions: T = negative 100°F and 15 inHg.

    A) 24.45 L
    B) 32.7 L
    C) 16.6 L
    D) 22.5 L

9. What is the molar volume of a gas at 300°C and 0.95 atm?

    A) 49.5 L
    B) 283 L
    C) 44 L
    D) 120 L

10. Disinfection means:

    A) Killing or removing all organisms.
    B) Using specialized cleansing techniques that destroy or prevent growth of organisms capable of infection.
    C) Halting the growth of all microorganisms.
    D) Removing microorganisms from other living organisms.

11. Which of the following statements is incorrect regarding universal precautions?

    A) Applies to all male and female bodily fluids, including urine, sweat, and breastmilk.
    B) Defined as an approach to infection control.
    C) Correct to treat all bodily fluids as though they are infectious.
    D) Employee uniforms do not necessarily serve as personal protective equipment or satisfy universal precautions.

12. With regard to airborne bioaerosol samples, viable and fungal counts are most accurate when taken:

    A) In complaint and non-complaint areas of the building, as well as outside of the building.
    B) Both on-site and in nearby buildings for reference.
    C) In complaint areas only.
    D) On hot days.

13. A set of 15 air samples was collected for measurement of exposure to total particulates. The results are 8.4 mg/m^3, 10.5 mg/m^3, 12.7 mg/m^3, 18.9 mg/m^3, 19.7 mg/m^3, 20.6 mg/m^3, 20.9 mg/m^3, 21.1 mg/m^3, 21.8 mg/m^3, and 22.3 mg/m^3.

    The data is presented in the table below.

Table: Total Particulate Exposure

X_i (mg/m^3)
8.4
10.5
12.7
18.9
19.7
20.6
20.9
21.1
21.8
22.3
24.9
25.1
25.7
26.0
29.6

Calculate the geometric mean (nth root form).

A) $12.34 \, mg/m^3$
B) $16.50 \, mg/m^3$
C) $19.52 \, mg/m^3$
D) $28.78 \, mg/m^3$

14. Suppose two methods are used to analyze for ammonia. An atmosphere of ammonia vapor in air is generated, and 15 samples are collected with method 1, and 12 samples with method 2. The following results are obtained:

Method 1: mean = 12.4 ppm, SD = 2.33 ppm, n = 15
Method 2: mean = 15.7 ppm, SD = 3.73 ppm, n = 12

Calculate the pooled standard deviation.

A) 3.12 ppm
B) 4.55 ppm
C) 5.10 ppm
D) 8.90 ppm

15. In order to assess how strongly related an exposure is to a disease, which would be the best health statistic?

A) Incidence of the disease among the exposed.
B) Attributable risk.
C) Prevalence of the exposure.
D) Relative risk.
E) Proportionate mortality.

16. An average flow rate of a stack is 1000 CFM and an average SO_2 concentration of 1000 ppm. What is the mass emission rate of SO_2 in pounds per hour?

A) 1 to 2 lb/hr.
B) 2 to 4 lb/hr.
C) 4 to 6 lb/hr.
D) Greater than 6 lb/hr.

17. An environmental engineer is testing your pollution control knowledge in a staff meeting. The site is reviewing a new process that will be emitting ammonia. Select the most appropriate air-cleaning device for ammonia.

A) Electrostatic precipitator.
B) Sand filter bed.
C) Absorber.
D) It is not possible to remove the ammonia from the air stream.

18. An exhaust fan was selected for a particular industrial process to exhaust 40,000 CFM against a system static pressure of 4.0 inches WG when operating at 1,600 RPM and developing 20 BHP. Upon installation, it was discovered that the fan was actually exhausting 50,000 CFM. Use the fan law(s) to calculate the new BHP developed.

RPM 2 = 1,280 RPM

A) 10.2 BHP
B) 12.4 BHP
C) 16.6 BHP
D) 18.8 BHP

19. A manometer took several readings on a fan's inlet and outlet sides. Calculate the fan static pressure (FSP) if the static pressure on the outlet side of the fan is 0.9 inches WG, static pressure on the inlet side of the fan is 3.2 inches WG, and the velocity pressure is 1.0 inches WG.

A) 2.5 inches WG
B) 3.1 inches WG
C) 3.9 inches WG
D) 4.8 inches WG

20. Calculate the hood static pressure when the duct velocity is 0.25 inches WG and the hood entry loss is 0.50 inches WG, assuming standard temperature and pressure.

A) 0.75 inches WG
B) 0.25 inches WG
C) 0.50 inches WG
D) 0.2 inches WG

21. Tenosynovitis is inflammation and swelling of the _____ frequently caused by repetitive movements.

A) Tendons.
B) Ligaments.
C) Cartilage.
D) Tenovium tissue.

22. Which of the following is not a work-related risk factor for musculoskeletal disorders?

A) Mechanical stress.
B) Posture.
C) Low temperatures.
D) Resonance.

23. What is the Recommended Weight Limit (RWL) for the following conditions?

- Weight to be lifted = 20 lbs
- Distance between body and hand grip on the object to be lifted = 24 inches
- Vertical position at the beginning of the lift = 36 inches
- Vertical position at end of lift = 46 inches
- Frequency of lift = once every 5 minutes for eight hours

Note: Hand coupling is poor and this job requires a twist from the "eyes front" position of 15°.

A) 14.8 lbs
B) 16.8 lbs
C) 20 lbs
D) 26.8 lbs

24. What is the appropriate method when sampling for Acetone?

A) OSHA 954.
B) NIOSH 1000.
C) NIOSH 1300.
D) OSHA 1450.

25. Given a measured value 20 ppm of methyl ethyl ketone with a TLV of 200 ppm, and 1 mg/m^3 of terephthalic acid with a TLV of 10 mg/m^3, calculate the total values.

A) 0.04
B) 0.20
C) 0.86
D) 1.22

26. An industrial hygienist conducted an 8-hour TWA sampling for acetone, ethyl acetate, and ethyl ether. See concentrations below:

- Acetone: 500 ppm
- Ethyl Acetate: 100 ppm
- Ethyl Ether: 110 ppm

Acetone's 8-hour TWA Permissible Exposure Limit (PEL) is 1,000 ppm. Ethyl Acetate's 8-hour TWA Permissible Exposure Limit (PEL) is 400 ppm. Ethyl Ether's 8-hour TWA Permissible Exposure Limit (PEL) is 400 ppm. What is the additive mixture exposure value for acetone, ethyl acetate, and ethyl ether, and does this value make the worker over exposed?

A) .15, the worker is not overexposed.
B) .88, the worker is not overexposed.
C) 1.025, the worker is overexposed.
D) 1.80, the worker is overexposed.

27. Which of the following is not an AIHA Management System Component?

    A) Responsibility and authority.
    B) Inspection and evaluation.
    C) Define leadership.
    D) Communication systems.

28. Instruments used for emergency response situations should be calibrated:

    A) Annually.
    B) Quarterly.
    C) Monthly.
    D) Before and after each emergency response.

29. Which of the following answers is not included in a Process Safety hazard analysis?

    A) Human factors.
    B) Quantitative proportion of employees and annual process injuries.
    C) Qualitative evaluation of failure of controls on employees.
    D) Facility siting.

30. In the corner of a large room, a machine is generating sound at a power level of 110 dB. Determine the estimated sound pressure level at a distance of 10 feet.

    A) 76 dB
    B) 82 dB
    C) 99 dB
    D) 109 dB

31. What is the frequency of sound in air if the wavelength is 30 cm?

    A) 978 Hz
    B) 1075 Hz
    C) 1147 Hz
    D) 1328 Hz

32. An industrial hygiene technician conducted sampling at a steel mill. The employee has an 8-hour TWA of 98 decibels. The hearing protection the employee was wearing has an NRR of 32 dB. Considering the employee is trained and using the hearing protection correctly, what is the employee's estimated noise exposure?

    A) 80 dBA
    B) 86 dBA
    C) 91 dBA
    D) 94 dBA

33. Workers must use respiratory protection due to the presence of harmful vapors in air despite the implementation of engineered controls that include ventilation. The elastomeric ½ face respirator that has been used for the previous three years has been discontinued by the manufacturer. After reviewing the available respirators, a different elastomeric ½ face respirator is selected. Best practice dictates that the following should be performed prior to issuing the new respirator to the workers.

    A) Collect the old respirators for redistribution.
    B) Fit-test the workers for the new respirator.
    C) Fit-test and train the workers for the new respirator.
    D) Fit-test, train and photograph the workers while wearing the new respirator.

34. An air-purifying respirator (APR) is utilized in which hazardous material PPE ensemble level?

    A) Level A
    B) Level B
    C) Level C
    D) Level D

35. Which statement is false in regards to quantitative fit testing?

    A) Measures fit factors greater than 10,000.
    B) Requires a probed face piece or probe adaptor.
    C) The fit test subject can provide a false response to the test.
    D) Fits any tight-fitting respirator.

36. A source is producing 125 mR/hour at 1 meter. Workers must perform repairs in the same room as the source but must not be exposed to more than 1 mR for the hour the repair task will require. What distance must be maintained from the source by the workers to prevent the exposure from being unacceptable during the task?

    A) 11.2 m
    B) 0.9 m
    C) 110 m
    D) 11 m

37. Health physics literature states that a short-term dose of 10 Gy is usually fatal. Calculate this dose in mrad.

    A) 1,000,000
    B) 10,000
    C) 1000
    D) 100

38. The half-life of Iodine-131 is 8.02 days. The biological half-life of iodine in the thyroid is approximately 115 days. The activity level of iodine in a person's thyroid on March 1 is 35 microcuries. What is the estimated activity level in the person's thyroid on April 1st?

    A) 0.45 microcuries
    B) 1.99 microcuries
    C) 5.59 microcuries
    D) 10.34 microcuries

39. To evaluate low frequency (<300 MHz) RF field exposure, it may be necessary to evaluate which of the following:

    A) Power density and specific absorption.
    B) Power density and induced currents.
    C) E&H field strength, induced current and contact current.
    D) Power density and contact current.

40. For non-ionizing radiation, energies with shorter wavelengths have magnetic fields that are:

    A) Perpendicular.
    B) Not perpendicular.
    C) Convex.
    D) Not convex.

41. Exposure to intense light from sources, including the sun, carbon arc, or welder's arc, without proper protection may produce what medical condition?

    A) Photoconjunctivitis.
    B) Retinal Scotomas "Blind Spots."
    C) Corneal Abrasion.
    D) Erythema.

42. What are the classic symptoms of heat stroke?

    A) Headache, nausea, dizziness.
    B) Weakness, fatigue.
    C) Elevated body temperature, loss of consciousness, hot dry skin.
    D) Excessive sweating, severe cramps.

43. If the work force is performing moderate work (350 kcal/hour), and the WBGT reading is 84.7°F, what is the designated work-rest regimen for an acclimatized worker based on the table shown below?

Work-Rest Regimen	Heavy Work	Moderate Work	Light Work
25% Work 75% Rest	30.0	31.1	32.2
50% Work 50% Rest	27.9	29.4	31.4
75% Work 25% Rest	27.9 25.9	29.4 28.0	30.6
Continuous	25.0	26.7	30.0

    A) 75% work – 25% rest
    B) 50% work – 50% rest
    C) 25% work – 75% rest
    D) Continuous work

44. What OSHA standard addresses heat stress within general industry?

    A) 1910.95
    B) 1910.178
    C) 1910.179
    D) Currently OSHA does not have a Heat Stress Standard

45. Death associated with repeated ingestion of warfarin, fumarin, and PMP is attributed to:

    A) Respiratory arrest.
    B) Internal hemorrhaging.
    C) Liver toxicity.
    D) CNS depression.

46. Which of the following agents is most likely to penetrate to the deep lung regions?

    A) Ammonia.
    B) Chlorine.
    C) Sulfur dioxide.
    D) Ozone.

47. Which of the following are the primary determinants for the occurrence of passive transport?

    A) Metabolic work, ionization of the compound.
    B) Pinocytosis, phagocytosis.
    C) A concentration gradient across membranes, liposolubility of the compound, ionization of the compound.
    D) Metabolic inhibition, receptor site competition.

48. Heating and melting solids results in the generation of fumes. Select the primary fume generated in iron and steel foundry operations.

    A) Hexavalent chromium.
    B) Crystalline silica.
    C) Iron oxide.
    D) Nickel.

49. An office building serves 100 occupants. The building HVAC system supplies 10,000 CFM. What is the outdoor air ventilation rate per person if the building HVAC system supplies 10,000 CFM, and 80% of the air is recirculated?

    A) 0 CFM/person.
    B) 10 CFM/person.
    C) 20 CFM/person.
    D) 30 CFM/person.

50. Choose the answer that is the predominant source of exposure during grinding processes.

    A) Particulates discharged from the grinder.
    B) Abrasives used in the grinding wheel.
    C) Abrasive bonding material.
    D) Heat generated from the grinder.

Self-Assessment Exam 1 Answers

1. Answer: D
   Explanation: When E has been determined, calculate the concentration, C (fibers/cc), of fibers in the air volume sampled, V (Liters), using the effective collection area of the filter, A_c (approx. 385 mm² for a 25-mm filter):

   The formula used to calculate the airborne concentration of fibers using fiber density (E):

   $$C_{asb} = \frac{EA_c}{(V)(10^3)}$$

   Where:
   C_{asb} is the airborne concentration of fibers in fibers/mL
   E is the fiber density in fibers/mm²
   A_c is the effective collection area of a filter (approximately 385 mm² for a 25 mm filter)
   V is the volume of sampled air in liters. In this example 450 minutes x 2 L/m = 900L

   $$C_{asb} = \frac{(381\frac{f}{mm^2})(385mm^2)}{(900L)(10^3\frac{mL}{L})}$$

   C_{asb} = 0.16 f/mL and since mL and cc are equivalent 0.16 f/cc

2. Answer: C
   Explanation: PEL = 400/10 PEL = 40 µg/m³
                            Source 29 CFR 1910.1025

3. Answer: D
   Explanation: The coulometric cell has a semipermeable membrane that selectively allows oxygen to enter the cell. The coulometric cell is also used for carbon monoxide detection. *Source: Fundamentals of Industrial Hygiene 6th ed. NSC*

4. Answer: A
   Explanation:
   $$1 \text{ atm} = 760 \text{ mmHg} = P_{total}$$

   $$P_{total} = P(N_2) + P(O_2) + P(CO_2)$$

5. Answer: A
   Explanation: According to the NIOSH Manual of Analytical Methods, the appropriate method when sampling for Vinyl Chloride is NIOSH 1007 – solid sorbent tubes (2 – tandem) and analyzed by gas chromatography + FID. *Source: NIOSH Manual of Analytical Methods 4th edition*

6. Answer: A

   Explanation: Benzo(a) pyrene is analyzed per NIOSH 5506 – HPLC fluorescence/UV. Oil mist on a PVC filter is analyzed per NIOSH 5206 – Infrared spectrophotometry. Nitrous Oxide in a bag is analyzed per NIOSH 6600 – Infrared spectrophotometry. Quartz (silica) on a PVC filter is analyzed per NIOSH 7603 – Infrared spectrophotometry. *Source: NIOSH Manual of Analytical Methods 4th edition*

7. Answer: C

   Explanation: The closer an object is to the eye, the more convex the human eye lens must become in order to focus on it. Through aging, the human lens loses its accommodative power (elasticity) and its power of thickening. This condition is known as presbyopia, and usually develops after age 40 years. *Source: Fundamentals of Industrial Hygiene 5th Edition*

8. Answer: B

   Explanation:

   Step 1: Convert temperature to absolute
   $$77°F + 460 = 537°R$$
   $$-100°F + 460 = 360°R$$

   Step 2: Calculate the molar volume under field conditions

   Use Ideal Gas Law to determine molar volume of field conditions

   $$\frac{P_1 V_1}{T_1} = \frac{P_2 V_2}{T_2}$$

   Note: All must be in absolute units

   $$\frac{29.92 inHg(24.45)}{537} = \frac{15 inHg(V_2)}{360}$$

   $$\frac{29.92 inHg(24.45)(360)}{537 x 15 inHg} = V_2$$

   $$V_2 = 32.7 \text{ L}$$

9. Answer: A

   Explanation:

   Step 1: Convert to absolute
   $$300°C + 273°C = 573°C$$

   Using the ideal gas law solve for V1

   $$\frac{V_1 x (P_1)}{T_1} = \frac{P_2 x V_2}{T_2}$$

   $$\frac{22.4 x (1)}{273} = \frac{.95 x V_2}{573}$$

$$V_2 = \frac{22.4\, x(573)}{273 x.95}$$

$$V_2 = 49.5\ \text{L}$$

10. Answer: B

    Explanation: Disinfection describes a process that eliminates many or all pathogenic microorganisms, except bacterial spores, on inanimate objects. *Source: CDC Guideline for Disinfection and Sterilization in Healthcare Facilities.*

11. Answer: A

    Explanation: Universal precautions apply to blood, fluids in which blood is indistinguishably mixed, and bodily fluids that visibly contain blood; however, the examples in answer "A" are excluded from universal precautions unless they visibly contain blood.

12. Answer: A

    Explanation: Currently, there are no regulations addressing fungal biohazard exposure levels. Accordingly, comparing sample results from the complaint area with results from non-complaint and outdoor areas provides information for decision making.

13. Answer: C

    Explanation:

Table: Geometric Mean (nth root form)

$X_i\ (mg/m^3)$
8.4
10.5
12.7
18.9
19.7
20.6
20.9
21.1
21.8
22.3
24.9
25.1
25.7
26.0
29.6

Calculate the geometric mean (nth root form)

$$GM = \sqrt[n]{(x_1)(x_2)\ldots(x_n)}$$

$$GM = \sqrt[15]{(8.4\ x\ 10.5\ x\ 12.7\ x\ 18.9\ x\ 19.7\ x\ 20.6\ x\ 20.9\ x\ 21.1\ x\ 21.8\ x\ 22.3\ x\ 24.9\ x\ 25.1\ x\ 25.7\ x\ 26.0\ x\ 29.6)}$$

$$GM = 19.52\ mg/m^3$$

Source: Industrial-Occupational Hygiene Calculations: A Professional Reference

14. Answer: A
    Explanation:
    Method 1: mean = 12.4 ppm, SD = 2.33 ppm, n = 15
    Method 2: mean = 15.7 ppm, SD = 3.73 ppm, n = 12

    Step 1: Calculate the SD_{pooled}

    $$SD_{pooled} = \sqrt{\frac{(n_1 - 1)SD_1{}^2 + (n_2 - 1)SD_2{}^2}{n_1 + n_2 - 2}}$$

    $$SD_{pooled} = \sqrt{\frac{(14)(2.33)^2 + (12)(3.73)^2}{25}}$$

    $$SD_{pooled} = 3.12 \; ppm$$

Source: Industrial-Occupational Hygiene Calculations: A Professional Reference

15. Answer D
    Explanation: Relative risk is defined as the ratio of the risk of disease in exposed individuals to the risk of disease in nonexposed individuals. Relative risk tells the assessor the size of the excess risk that the subject with exposure to a factor runs, compared with a subject without exposure to such a factor. Relative risk identifies subjects at a high risk of certain outcomes. The relative risk measures the strength of an association; thus, a high relative risk suggests etiology or causality. *Source: Epidemiology 5th Edition, Leon Gordis*

16. Answer: D
    Explanation:

    Step 1: Calculate the mass of emission assuming Normal Temperature and Pressure

    $$MW \; of \; SO_2 = 32 + 2(16) = 64$$

    $$mg/m^3 = \frac{ppm \; x \; mw}{24.45}$$

    $$mg/m^3 = \frac{1000(64)}{24.45} = 2{,}617 \; mg/m^3$$

    Step 2: Convert mg/m^3 to $pounds/m^3$

    $$2{,}617 \; mg/m^3 \; x \; \frac{g}{1000 \; mg} \; x \; \frac{lb}{454 \; g} = 0.006 \; lb/m^3$$

    Step 3: Convert CFM to m^3/hr

$$\frac{1000\ ft^3}{min} \ x \ \frac{m^3}{35.3\ ft^3} \ x \ \frac{60\ min}{hr} = 1700 \ m^3/hr$$

Step 4: Calculate the pounds per hour

$$\frac{0.006\ lb}{m^3} \ x \ \frac{1700\ m^3}{hr} = 10 \ lb/hr$$

Single calculation method:

$$\frac{1000\ FT^3}{min} \ x \ \frac{60\ min}{hr} \ x \ \frac{2,617\ mg}{m^3} \ x \ \frac{m^3}{35.3\ FT^3} \ x \ \frac{lb}{454\ gm} \ x \ \frac{gm}{1000\ mg} = 9.8 \ lb/hr$$

Note: Difference due to rounding

17. Answer: C
    Explanation: The electrostatic precipitator and sand filter are better choices for particulates. Absorbers are used for removing gasses from air streams. *Source: Air Pollution Control Engineering, 2nd Edition*

18. Answer: A
    Explanation:

$$\frac{BHP\ 1}{BHP\ 2} = \left(\frac{RPM\ 1}{RPM2}\right)^3$$

$$\frac{20}{BHP\ 2} = \left(\frac{1,600}{1,280}\right)^3$$

$$BHP\ 2 = \frac{20}{\left(\frac{1,600}{1,280}\right)^3}$$

$$BHP\ 2 = 10.2\ BHP$$

19. Answer: B
    Explanation:

$$FSP = SP_{out} - SP_{in} - VP_{in}$$

$$Sp_{out} = 0.9\ inches\ WG$$
$$SP_{in} = 3.2\ inches\ WG$$
$$VP_{in} = 1.0\ inches\ WG$$

Step 1: Solve for FSP

$$FSP = SP_{out} - SP_{in} - VP_{in}$$

$$FSP = 0.9\ inches\ WG - (-3.2\ inches\ WG) - 1.0\ inches\ WG$$
$$FSP = 3.1\ inches\ WG$$

20. Answer: A
    Explanation:

$$SPh = VP + He$$

$$SPh = 0.25 + 0.50$$

$$SPh = 0.75 \text{ inches WG}$$

Laboratory Ventilation Workbook, Burton

21. Answer: A
    Explanation: It is the inflammation of the synovium, the fluid filled sheath of tendons. *Source: The Occupational Environment, Its Evaluation, Control, and Management. 3rd edition*

22. Answer: D
    Explanation: Resonance is the quality of sound. All other answer choices are related to musculoskeletal disorders. *Source: The Occupational Environment, Its Evaluation, Control, and Management. 3rd edition*

23. Answer: A
    Explanation: The 1991 NIOSH lifting equation is a specialized risk assessment tool. It has been designed to meet selected lifting related criteria and encompasses biomechanical, work physiology, and psychophysical elements in a practical application framework that, if followed, will result in a reduced number of work place mishaps.

$$RWL = LC \times HM \times VM \times DM \times AM \times FM \times CM$$

$$RWL = 51\left(\tfrac{10}{H}\right)(1 - .0075\,|\,V\text{-}30\,|)\left(.82 + \tfrac{1.8}{D}\right)\left(1 - (0.0032 \times A)\right)(FM)(CM)$$

$$RWL = 51\left(\tfrac{10}{24}\right)(1 - .0075 \times 6)\left(.82 + \tfrac{1.8}{10}\right)\left(1 - (0.0032 \times 15)\right)(0.85)(0.9)$$

$$RWL = 51 \times 0.417 \times .955 \times 1 \times 0.952 \times 0.85 \times 0.9$$

$$RWL = 14.8 \text{ lbs}$$

24. Answer: C
    Explanation: According to the NIOSH Manual of Analytical Methods, the appropriate method when sampling for acetone is NIOSH 1300, the Ketone I method. The method specifies a solid sorbent tube (coconut shell) and analysis by gas chromatography-FID. The carrier gas is listed as either nitrogen or helium. *Source: NIOSH Manual of Analytical Methods 4th edition*

25. Answer: B

   Explanation: Workplace atmospheric mixtures also may be comprised of agents with different toxicological effects and target organs. That is, the effects are not considered to be additive. The exposure assessment is simpler but still uses the acceptable total value of 1.0.

$$TV_1 = \frac{C_1}{TLV_1}$$

$$TV_2 = \frac{C_2}{TLV_2}$$

$$TV_n = \frac{C_n}{TLV_n}$$

Step 1: Solve for the total value for condition 1

$$TV_1 = \frac{C_1}{TLV_1}$$

$$TV_1 \, methyl \, ethyl \, ketone = \frac{20}{200}$$

$$TV_1 \, methyl \, ethyl \, ketone = 0.1$$

Step 2: Solve for the total value for condition 2

$$TV_2 = \frac{C_2}{TLV_2}$$

$$TV_2 \, terephthalic \, acid = \frac{1}{10}$$

$$TV_2 \, terephthalic \, acid = 0.1$$

Since each condition is less than 1.0, it could be concluded from this evaluation that the exposures may not have exceeded the acceptable limits. *Source: The Occupational Environment: Its Evaluation, Control and Management 3rd edition, Volume 1*

26. Answer: C

   Explanation:

   Step 1: Use the Additive Mixture Formula

$$\frac{C_1}{T_1} + \frac{C_2}{T_2} \cdots \frac{C_n}{T_n}$$

$$\frac{500 \, ppm}{1,000 \, ppm} + \frac{100 \, ppm}{400 \, ppm} + \frac{110 \, ppm}{400 \, ppm} = .50 + .25 + .275 = 1.025$$

Since the unity is greater than 1.0, the worker is overexposed due to the additive mixture effect.
Source: TLVs and BEIS Based on the Documentation of the Threshold Limit Values for Chemical Substances and Physical Agents & Biological Exposure Indices.

27. Answer: C
Explanation: AIHA lists the following components of Management System Criteria:

Component	Description/Objective
Health and safety policy	States organizational health and safety objectives, and helps to ensure top management commitment.
Responsibility and authority	Ensures that all members of an organization are accountable for health and safety issues and understand their roles and responsibilities, while having accountability for their actions.
Resources	Seeks to ensure that organizations are sufficiently funded to adequately address health and safety issues.
Written documentation	Develops a manual that documents all components that organization will employ to adhere to the management system requirements.
Procedures	Establishes operational procedures detailing the recognition, evaluation, and control of health and safety hazards in the workplace.
Planning	Assessments should be conducted to evaluate deficiencies and establish corrective intervention strategies.
Compliance and conformance review	Defines and documents procedures to ensure a process exists to stay abreast of pending/current legislation/regulation and develops appropriate organizational responses accordingly.
Goals and objectives	Establishes health and safety objectives and verifies success of the objectives through key metrics, such as accident/injury rates, and illness rates.
Design control	Establishes and maintains procedures to ensure that workstations are designed in a manner to control potential hazards, both health and safety scope.
Document and data control	Develops and implements procedures to ensure management of all elements related to health and safety documentation.
Purchasing	Establishes procedures to evaluate potential toxicological impact associated with product purchase for the organization, as well as adequately ensuring contractor adherence to health and safety stipulations.
Communication systems	Develops and implements procedures to communicate critical health and safety requirements to employees and contractors in a timely manner to prevent and minimize hazards and potential exposures.
Inspection and evaluation	Establishes protocols to routinely inspect/audit the workplace for health and safety deficiencies
Corrective and preventive action	Establishes procedures to implement corrective actions and procedures.
Training	Ensure that employees are provided with appropriate training to educate them of the hazards of the workplace, while adhering to all regulatory requirements related to training.

28. Answer: D

Explanation: If an emergency response occurs, instrumentation used in the emergency response should be calibrated before each use to verify accuracy and function. Calibration after each emergency response situation allows for identification of faulty equipment and prepares the instrument for quick turn-around. ISEA updated its position statement on instrument calibration in 2010, stating, "A bump test . . . or calibration check of portable gas monitors should be conducted before each day's use in accordance with the manufacturer's instructions." If an instrument fails a bump test or a calibration check, the operator should perform a full calibration on it before using it. If the instrument fails the full calibration, the employer should remove it from service. *Source: www.osha.gov*

29. Answer: B

Explanation: The following are parts involved in a process safety hazard analysis: facility siting, human factors, and qualitative evaluation of failure of controls on employees. *Source: www.osha.gov*

30. Answer: C

Explanation:

$$L_P = L_W - 20 \log r - 0.5 + DI + T$$

T is the correction factor to temperature and pressure (assumed to be zero)

$$L_W = 110 \, dB$$
$$r = 10 \, feet$$
$$DI = 10 \log Q$$
$$Q = 8 \, (because \, of \, a \, room \, corner$$
$$T = 0$$

Step 1: Solve for DI

$$DI = 10 \log 8$$
$$DI = 9.03$$

Step 2: Solve for L_P

$$L_P = 110 - 20 \log 10 - 0.5 + 9.03 + 0$$

$$L_P = 99 \, dB$$

Source: Source: Industrial-Occupational Hygiene Calculations: A Professional Reference

31. Answer: C
   Explanation:

$$f = \frac{c}{\lambda}$$

Step 1: Solve for f

$$f = \frac{344\,\frac{m}{sec}}{0.3m}$$

$$f = 1147\,Hz$$

Source: Occupational Safety Calculations: A Professional Reference, 2nd edition

32. Answer: B
Explanation: Noise Reduction Ratings are found in the OSHA Technical Manual. When OSHA promulgated its Hearing Conservation Amendment in 1983, it incorporated the EPA labeling requirements for hearing protectors (40 CFR 211), which required manufacturers to identify the noise reduction capability of all hearing protectors on the hearing protector package. This measure is referred to as the noise reduction rating (NRR). It is a laboratory derived numerical estimate of the attenuation achieved by the protector. It became apparent that the amount of actual protection in the workplace with the designated hearing protectors did not correlate with the attenuation indicated by the NRR. OSHA acknowledged that in most cases, this number overstated the protection afforded to workers and required the application for certain circumstances of a safety factor of 50% to the NRR, above and beyond the 7 dB subtraction called for when using A-weighted measurements.

For example, consider a worker who is exposed to 98 dBA for 8 hours and whose hearing protectors have an NRR of 25 dB. We can estimate the worker's resultant exposure using the 50% safety factor. The worker's resultant exposure is 89 dBA in this case.

The 50% safety factor adjusts labeled NRR values for workplace conditions and is used when considering whether engineering controls are to be implemented.

$$Estimated\ dBA\ exposure = TWA(dBA) - [(25 - 7)\ x\ 50\%] = 89\ dBA$$

Though using the 50% safety factor produces the most reliable result, it is not used for enforcement purposes. For enforcement purposes, CSHOs should subtract 7 dB from the NRR without considering the 50% safety factor.

Rewriting the above formula to divide by 2 rather than multiply by 50%:

$$Estimated\ Noise\ Exposure = TWA - \left(\frac{NRR - 7}{2}\right)$$

Step 1: Solve for Estimated Noise Exposure

$$Estimated\ Noise\ Exposure = 98 - \left(\frac{32 - 7}{2}\right)$$

$$Estimated\ Noise\ Exposure = 98 - 12.5$$

$$Estimated\ Noise\ Exposure = 86\ dBA$$

Source: OSHA Technical Manual

33. Answer: C

Explanation: Fit-test and training are critical requirements. A photograph is not of significant value. The workers must also demonstrate the ability to properly use the new respirator. *Source: Industrial Hygiene Reference and Study Guide, 3rd edition*

34. Answer: C

Explanation: Personal protective equipment is divided into four categories based on the degree of protection afforded. *Level A* is selected when the greatest level of skin, respiratory, and eye protection is required. Level A respirator protection includes a positive pressure, full face-piece self-contained breathing apparatus (SCBA), or positive pressure supplied air respirator with escape SCBA, approved by NIOSH. *Level B* is the highest level of respiratory protection necessary but a lesser level of skin protection is needed. Level B respirator protection includes a positive pressure, full face-piece self-contained breathing apparatus (SCBA), or positive pressure supplied air respirator with escape SCBA, approved by NIOSH. *Level C* is to be used when the concentration(s) and type(s) of airborne substance(s) is known and the criteria for using air-purifying respirators are met. Level C respirator protection includes a full-face or half-mask, air purifying respirators approved by NIOSH. *Level D* uses no respiratory protection. *OSHA 1910.120 App B; osha.gov*

35. Answer: C

Explanation: Portacount fit testing is utilized for quantitative fit testing, and it is possible to measure a fit factor greater than 10,000.

Advantages of quantitative fit testing: No protection-factor limit, documentation of numerical results, eliminates chance of employee deception or bluffing.

Disadvantages of quantitative fit testing: Expensive up-front equipment costs, requires probed face-piece or probe adapter, and annual recalibration of equipment is suggested.

OSHA recognizes three types of quantitative fit testing protocol agents: generated aerosol, ambient aerosol condensation nuclei count (CNC), and controlled negative pressure (CNP). All three types of quantitative fit testing use a digital instrument that measures airborne particles inside and outside the test respirator or measures vacuum pressure. A special sampling probe takes measurements inside the mask. *Sources: tsi.com and OSHA.gov*

36. Answer: A
    Explanation: The task will take 1 hour so the unit of time for the exposure is equivalent.

    Step 1: Use the inverse square law to solve for the distance

    $$\frac{I_1}{I_2} = \left[\frac{d_2}{d_1}\right]^2$$

    $$\frac{1.25\ mr/Hr}{1\ mR/Hr} = \left[\frac{d_2}{1\ meter}\right]^2$$

    $$\sqrt{1.25x1\ m^2} = d_2$$

    $$11.2\ m = d_2$$

    Rounding down to 11 would allow the dose to exceed 1 mR per hour; therefore, use 11.2 or round up to 12 if 11.2 is not a choice.

37. Answer: A
    Explanation:

    1Gray = 100 rad, therefore 10 Gray x100 rad/Gray x 1000 mrad/rad = 1000000 mrad
    Source: The Occupational Environment: Its Evaluation, Control and Management, 3rd Edition

38. Answer: B
    Explanation:
    Step 1: Determine the effective half-life of Iodine-131 in the thyroid

    $$T_{\frac{1}{2}eff} = \frac{\left(T_{\frac{1}{2}rad}\right)\left(T_{\frac{1}{2}bio}\right)}{T_{\frac{1}{2}rad} + T_{\frac{1}{2}bio}}$$

    $$T_{\frac{1}{2}eff} = \frac{(8.02\ days)(115\ days)}{8.02\ days + 115\ days}$$

    $$T_{\frac{1}{2}eff} = 7.50\ days$$

Step 2: Determine the activity level after 31 days

$$A = A_i (0.5)^{\frac{t}{T_{\frac{1}{2}}}}$$

$$A = 35\ \mu C (0.5)^{\frac{31}{7.50}}$$

$$A = 1.99\ \mu C$$

Source: None provided

39. Answer: C

Explanation: The Specific Absorption Rate (SAR) is fundamental to exposure criteria. In free fields, power density, electric field strength, and magnetic field strength are considered. Power density is most meaningful at frequencies above 300 MHz while guidelines require the evaluation of both E and H fields at frequencies less than 300 MHz. E is the electric field strength (V/m) and H is the magnetic field strength (A/m). *Sources: (1) Applications and Computational Elements of Industrial Hygiene, Stern and Mansdorf. (2) ACGIH Threshold Limit Values for Chemical Substances and Physical Agents 2015.*

40. Answer: A

Explanation: Non-ionizing radiation have wavelengths that are perpendicular.
Source: Industrial Hygiene Reference and Study Guide; Fleeger & Lillquist

41. Answer: B

Explanation: Exposure to intense light from sources such as the sun, carbon arc, or welder's arc without proper protection may produce temporary or permanent retinal scotomas (blind spots). Factors affecting the degree of retinal hazard include the size, type and spectral intensity of the source, the pupil size, retinal image quality, the spectral transmittance of the ocular media, the spectral adsorption of the retina and choroid, and the exposure duration. *Source: The Occupational Environment: Its Evaluation, Control, and Management 3rd Edition Volume 2*

42. Answer: C

Explanation: Headache, nausea, dizziness, weakness and fatigue are symptoms of heat exhaustion. Elevated body temperature, loss of consciousness, hot/dry skin, and convulsions are symptoms of heat stroke, which is a medical emergency. *Source: Applications and Computational Elements of Industrial Hygiene, Stern and Mansdorf*

43. Answer: B

   Explanation:

Work-Rest Regimen	Heavy Work	Moderate Work	Light Work
25% Work 75% Rest	30.0	31.1	32.2
50% Work 50% Rest	27.9	29.4	31.4
75% Work 25% Rest	27.9 25.9	29.4 28.0	30.6
Continuous	25.0	26.7	30.0

First, you must convert 84.7 °F to °C.   °C = (°F – 32) x 5/9   °C = 29.3
Looking at the table in the moderate work column, determine that 29.3 is between the 75% work temperature and 50% work temperature; therefore, choose the 50% work regimen.

44. Answer: D
   Explanation: Currently OSHA does not have a standard that deals specifically with heat stress. Citations for heat stress related matters generally come under the section 5(a)1 of the Occupational Safety and Health Act of 1970, which is better known as the "General Duty Clause."

45. Answer: B
   Explanation: These substances are anticoagulants, and death occurs following internal hemorrhaging.

46. Answer: D
   Explanation: Ozone is less water soluble and therefore more likely to penetrate further into the lungs.

47. Answer: C
   Explanation: All of the incorrect answers are associated with active transport.

48. Answer: C
   Explanation: Hexavalent chromium and nickel may be present, but in much smaller amounts than iron oxide. Crystalline silica is a dust and not a fume. *Source: Foundry Health Hazards publication, NOHSC, Government of Australia; and University of Utah lecture*

49. Answer: C

Explanation:

Step 1: Determine the amount of outdoor air

$$10,000\ CFM\ x\ 0.2 = 2,000\ CFM$$

Step 2: Determine the CFM per person

$$CFM\ per\ person = \frac{2,000\ CFM}{100\ people}$$

$$CFM\ per\ person = 20$$

Source: None

50. Answer: A

Explanation: The predominant source of exposure during grinding processes are particulates discharged from the grinder.

Self-Assessment Exam 2

1. The analytical method indicates the minimum volume is 10 Liters and the maximum volume is 100 Liters. The industrial hygienist believes the airborne concentration for the contaminant of interest is low and wants to obtain the lowest limit of detection possible per the method. The sample rate for the method is 0.5 L/m. What is the desired sample time?

   A) 480 minutes.
   B) 960 minutes.
   C) 200 minutes.
   D) 50 minutes.

2. A 200 mL burette is being used to calibrate the flow rate of a pump. The soap bubble travels from zero to 200 mL in 19.8 seconds. Calculate the flow rate for the pump.

   A) 1000 mL/min
   B) 2.0 L/min
   C) 0.6 mL/min
   D) 1000 cc/min

3. Choose the statement that best describes a TLV-time-weighted average (TWA).

   A) The time-weighted average concentration for a workday exceeding 4 hours that nearly all workers may be exposed to repeatedly for a working lifetime without adverse health effect.

   B) The average concentration for a workday that some workers may be exposed to repeatedly for a working lifetime without adverse health effect.

   C) The time-weighted average concentration for an 8-hour workday and a 40-hour workweek that nearly all workers may be exposed to repeatedly for a working lifetime without adverse health effect.

   D) The total-weighted average concentration for a workday exceeding 4 hours that nearly all workers may be exposed to repeatedly for a working lifetime without adverse health effect.

4. X-ray fluorescence is a technique that analyzes the radiation emitted from the contaminant after exposure to x-rays. This technique is utilized for which of the following?

   A) Crystals in tissue analysis.
   B) Lead wipe sample analysis.
   C) Hydrocarbons in exhaled air.
   D) Halogens in urine.

5. When conducting sampling for the alcohol Cyclohexanol, what is the recommended media?

   A) Solid Sorbent tube.
   B) 1 μm PTFE filter.
   C) 5 μm Preweighed PVC filter.
   D) Silica Gel Tube.

6. Convert 65°F to Centigrade.

   A) 18.3
   B) 4.1
   C) 25
   D) 33

7. Viral labyrinthitis and Meniere's Disease affect the vestibular system. What are the major symptoms?

   A) Loss of balance, vertigo, and nausea.
   B) Loss of balance, loss of hearing, and nausea.
   C) Sharp pain, vertigo, and loss of hearing.
   D) Sharp pain, loss of hearing, and nausea.

8. An IH trained in phase contrast microscopy is analyzing a filter for airborne asbestos fiber concentration. The sample for asbestos was collected over 450 minutes of an 8-hour shift at 2 L/m. After counting 100 fields, the average fiber count is 3 fibers per field. The field blank contains 0.01 fibers per field. It is known that the area of a 25 mm filter is 385 mm^2, and that the area of a graticule field is approximately 0.00785 mm^2. What is the fiber density, and is the sample acceptable?

   A) 147 f/mL or 147 f/cc
   B) 0.33 f/mL or 0.33 f/cc
   C) 1 f/mL or 1 f/cc
   D) 0.16 f/mL or 0.16 f/cc

9. 12.5 ml of a standard solution of 0.15 NHCl is used for titrating against NaOH using phenolphthalein. How many grams of NaOH were in the sample?

   A) 0.0037
   B) 0.074
   C) 0.037
   D) 0.00074

10. The use of chemicals or soaps to remove microbes from the skin or living tissue is best described as:

    A) Sterilization.
    B) Antisepsis.
    C) Disinfection.
    D) Decontamination.

11. Which of these methods is considered the "standard" for sampling airborne microorganisms?

    A) Petri dish.
    B) Membrane filter.
    C) The breather test.
    D) Multistage sieve impactor.

12. Blastomycosis is an infection caused by *Blastomyces. Blastomyces* is a _____.

   A) Virus.
   B) Fungi.
   C) Bacteria.
   D) Protozoa.

13. A study was conducted among a group of employees at Company XYZ to evaluate exposure to Acetone. The table represents eight Acetone exposure levels. The mean is 10.40 ppm.

Table: Acetone Exposure

Employee	Acetone Exposure (ppm)
1	15.9
2	20.6
3	11.9
4	4.1
5	2.5
6	7.5
7	12.3
8	8.4

Calculate the variance using the Acetone exposure table.

   A) 12.5 ppm^2
   B) 36.4 ppm^2
   C) 58.0 ppm^2
   D) 98.4 ppm^2

14. Choose the statement that best describes the median.

   A) The value in a set of measurements that occurs most frequently; the maximum value of a continuous probability density function.
   B) The positive square root of the variance of a distribution; the parameter measuring spread of values about the mean. It can be estimated from the slope of the straight line through data plotted on probability paper.
   C) The exposure measurement that divides a set of measurements into two equal parts, with half less than and half greater than this value.
   D) The difference between the largest and smallest values in a measurement data set.

15. In 1945, 1,000 women worked in a factory painting radium dials on watches. The incidence of bone cancer in these women up to 1975 was compared with that of 1,000 women who worked as telephone operators in 1945. Twenty of the radium dial workers and four of the telephone operators developed bone cancer between 1945 and 1975. The relative risk of developing bone cancer for radium dial workers is:

A) 2
B) 4
C) 5
D) 8

16. The following pollution controls operate by driving particulates to a wall or surface where they agglomerate into sand-like masses for collection and disposal:

A) Gravity settling chambers, cyclones, and electrostatic precipitators
B) Gravity settling chambers, depth filters, surface filters
C) Cyclones, surface filters, venturi scrubber
D) Depth filter, surface filter, venturi scrubber

17. What are the best actions to take to deal with pollutants?

A) Prevention and dispersion.
B) Dispersion, collection, and disposal.
C) Prevention and disposal.
D) Prevention, dispersion, collection, and disposal.

18. According to the US EPA, tropospheric ozone is formed when sunlight reacts with the following in the atmosphere.

A) Oxides of nitrogen, volatile organic compounds.
B) Oxides of sulfur, oxides of nitrogen.
C) Chlorine, fluorine.
D) Carbon monoxide, carbon dioxide, carbon disulfide.

19. A fan selected to operate at 9000 CFM, 1,500 RPM, requires 5 BHP at 1-inch WG. After installation, the process required an additional 2,000 CFM of air to make production target. Using the fan law(s), calculate the new speed, pressure, and brake horsepower requirements.

A) 1560 RPM, 1.5 inches WG, 6.5 BHP
B) 1650 RPM, 1.6 inches WG, 7.7 BHP
C) 1833 RPM, 1.5 inches WG, 9.1 BHP
D) 1833 RPM, 3.2 inches WG, 10.8 BHP

20. What is the velocity of air flowing through a 12-inch diameter duct if the velocity pressure in the duct is 3.8 inches WG?

A) 1009 FPM
B) 4532 FPM
C) 6711 FPM
D) 7807 FPM

21. What is the final room concentration of acetone if the vapor is generated at a rate of 8 CFM while the room is being ventilated with dilution air containing 40 PPM of acetone at a flow of 2,700 CFM?

    A) 3,003 PPM
    B) 4,653 PPM
    C) 5,908 PPM
    D) 8,851 PPM

22. The condition associated with irritation of the levator scapulae and the trapezius muscle group, commonly occurring after prolonged overhead work, is known as:

    A) Thoracic Outlet Syndrome.
    B) Neck Tension Syndrome.
    C) Raynaud's Syndrome.
    D) Frozen shoulder.

23. Which of the following is not a work-related risk factor for musculoskeletal disorders of the lower back?

    A) Anatomy.
    B) Asymmetrical handling.
    C) Repetition.
    D) Handles/coupling.

24. Calculate the RWL given the following conditions:

    - Weight to be lifted = 30 lbs (13.6 kg)
    - Distance between body and hand grip on the object to be lifted = 18 inches (45 cm)
    - Vertical position at the beginning of the lift = 30 inches (75 cm)
    - Vertical position at end of lift = 40 inches (100 cm)
    - Frequency of lift = once every 5 minutes for one hour.

    Note: Hand coupling is good, and this activity does not require any twisting movement.

    A) 14.0 kg
    B) 12.1 kg
    C) 13.6 kg
    D) 12.8 kg

25. Hazard is best described as:

    A) The source of risk.
    B) An assessment of vulnerability.
    C) A natural or manufactured event that has potential for harm.
    D) A function of vulnerability and risk.

26. Convert 10 ppm of Methylene chloride to milligrams per cubic meter. Reference information:
    Methylene chloride: CH_2Cl_2 Atomic Mass: C = 12, H = 1 & Cl = 35.5

    A) 11.9
    B) 20.5
    C) 34.7
    D) 70.5

27. An optical microscope is in use with the following conditions. The light source has a specified wavelength of 450 nm. The slide is viewed through water. The desired limit of resolution is 0.20 μm. According to the literature, the sine of an angle for this microscope is 0.97. Calculate the theoretical limit of resolution.

    A) 0.20 μm
    B) 2.0 μm
    C) 210 μm
    D) 213 nm

28. Which of the following are Environmental, Health, and Safety tools involved in the EHS Critical Process Interaction?

    A) Communicating, forecasting, guidance.
    B) Guidance, contracts.
    C) Business, community, company.
    D) Cross-functional management, critical requirements, communicating.

29. Select the best definition of leadership in an occupational setting.

    A) An inherent quality of the individual.
    B) The ability to mobilize available resources toward achieving organizational goals.
    C) The use of force to suppress dissent.
    D) A competitive winner.

30. Calculate the error of measurement if the true value is 20 ppm and the experimental value is 25 ppm.

    A) – 20%
    B) – 25%
    C) 20%
    D) 25%

31. An industrial hygienist conducted noise exposure sampling on an employee during a shift. The noise exposure sampling results are presented in the table below.

Average dBA	90	92	86	84
C_i	2	1	3	2

Calculate the percent dose for the employee during an 8-hour shift.

A) 70.6 dB
B) 73.5 dB
C) 84.0 dB
D) 91.3 dB

32. A worker at a manufacturing company is monitored for noise exposure. The results state that the worker had a dose of 150%. What is the TWA exposure?

A) 87 dBA
B) 93 dBA
C) 99 dBA
D) 102 dBA

33. Select the preferred method of noise control.

A) Path interruption.
B) Reduction at the receiver.
C) Reduction at the source.
D) Worker rotation.

34. Some of the requirements of ANSI Z87.1 are testing, normal, high-velocity and mass impact, penetration, flammability resistance, ease of cleaning, and minimum thickness. The ANSI document is related to:

A) Foot protection.
B) Hearing protection.
C) Head protection.
D) Eye and face protection.

35. Choose the class of hard hat that should be used to provide protection from falling objects and electrical shock from low voltages.

A) Class A.
B) Class C.
C) Class E.
D) Class G.

36. What factor listed below is the least likely to affect the cartridge life of respirator chemical cartridges?

    A) Relative humidity.
    B) Work rate.
    C) Workplace temperature.
    D) Chemical concentration.

37. Ionizing radiation is electromagnetic or particulate radiation that has enough energy to remove an electron from its orbit around the nucleus. Select the term that best describes the process in which energy moves the electron further away from the nucleus without removing it from orbit.

    A) Ionization.
    B) Photon mitigation.
    C) Neutronization.
    D) Excitation.

38. Select the radiation source material found in ceramic glazes and was used in the popular line of dinnerware known as 'Fiesta-Ware.'

    A) Thorium.
    B) Uranium.
    C) Cesium.
    D) Polonium.

39. Cesium-137 is a radioactive isotope material that has a half-life of 30.17 years, and the gamma ray constant is 2.60 R-cm^2/mCi-hr. The activity of the source is 3 microcuries. Estimate the radiation dose from the cesium-137 during a 3-hour exposure at a distance of approximately 20 feet from the source.

    A) 0.029 microREM
    B) 0.063 microREM
    C) 12.9 microREM
    D) 36.1 milliREM

40. Acute skin effects of exposure to UV in the 300 nm wavelength range include which of the following?

    A) Erythema, photosensitization.
    B) Melanosome expectoration.
    C) Premature aging.
    D) Hair movement, shock, burns.

41. The main UV source is the sun. Global UV radiation has two components. What are the components?

    A) Global temperature and sun's beam.
    B) Sky radiation and global temperature.
    C) Global temperature and global atmosphere conditions.
    D) Sun's beam and sky radiation.

42. As frequency increases, the wavelength decreases as you progress through the spectrum. Longer wavelengths are more penetrating to the body. Which of the following has the greatest ability to penetrate?

    A) UV.
    B) IR.
    C) Microwave.
    D) Blue light.

43. Which of the following lists the primary methods of heat transfer?

    A) Radiation, convection, conduction.
    B) Hot to cold objects.
    C) Evaporation, condensation.
    D) Solar, desalinization.

44. Assume wind speed is 5.8 m/sec and air temperature is 40°C, calculate the convective heat exchange.

    A) $48.7 \frac{kcal}{hr}$
    B) $65.0 \frac{kcal}{hr}$
    C) $83.1 \frac{kcal}{hr}$
    D) $100.5 \frac{kcal}{hr}$

$$C = 7.0 \, V_{air}^{0.6} (t_{air} - t_{skin})$$

Where:
C = Convective heat exchange, kcal/hour
V_{air} = Air velocity, meters per second
t_{air} = Air temperature, °C
t_{skin} = Mean weighted skin temperature (often assumed to be 35°C)

45. Which of the following can cause damage to bone marrow following prolonged exposure?

    A) Carbon dioxide.
    B) Lead.
    C) Toluene Diisocyanate.
    D) Beryllium.

46. Carbon monoxide is best described as:

    A) A pulmonary asphyxiant.
    B) A chemical asphyxiant.
    C) A simple asphyxiant.
    D) An irritant.

47. Which of the following is typical of methemoglobinemia?

    A) Heme iron is oxidized from ferrous to ferril state.
    B) Heme iron is oxidized from ferril to ferrous state.
    C) Heme iron is reduced from ferril to ferrous.
    D) Occurs only in vitro.

48. Natural gas and liquefied petroleum gasses are colorless and odorless. To improve detection of the presence of these flammable gases, an odorizing agent is added. Select the common odorizing agent:

    A) Ethyl mercaptan.
    B) Sulfur dioxide.
    C) Hydrogen sulfide.
    D) Sulfur trioxide.

49. Which of the following office indoor air pollution sources has the potential of being lethal to employees?

    A) Biological agents.
    B) Formaldehyde.
    C) Carbon dioxide.
    D) Poor ventilation.

50. Pot room workers in an aluminum smelter have developed an increase in bone density and irritation of the eyes and respiratory tract. What material is the likely cause of these effects?

    A) Fluoride.
    B) Sodium hydroxide.
    C) Nickel oxide.
    D) Osmic acid.

Self-Assessment Exam 1 Answers

1. Answer: C
   Explanation: Flow Rate x Time = Volume
   To obtain the lowest limit of detection, target the maximum Volume.

   0.5 L/m x Time = 100 L $Time = \dfrac{100\ L}{0.5\ L/m}$ Time = 200 minutes

2. Answer: C
   Explanation:

   $$200\ mL/19.8\ sec = 10.5\ mL/sec$$

   $$\frac{10.5\ mL}{sec} \ x \ \frac{60\ sec}{min} \ x \ \frac{1\ L}{1000\ mL} = 0.63\ \text{L/min}$$

3. Answer: C
   Explanation: The TWA concentration for a conventional 8-hour workday and a 40-hour workweek, to which it is believed that nearly all workers may be repeatedly exposed, day after day, for a working lifetime without adverse effect. Although calculating the average concentration for a workweek, rather than a workday, may be appropriate in some instances, ACHIH does not offer guidance regarding such exposures. *Source: TLVs and BEIs Based on Documentation of the Threshold Limit Values for Chemical Substances and Physical Agents & Biological Exposure Indices*

4. Answer: B
   Explanation: According to NIOSH publications, portable XRF can provide useful quantitative data for onsite risk assessment and clearance decisions for lead wipe samples. NIOSHTIC 20043982.

5. Answer: A
   Explanation: According to the NIOSH Manual of Analytical Methods, method 1402, the recommended media when sampling for Cyclohexanol is a solid sorbent tube (coconut shell). The analysis is done via gas chromatography-FID.
   Source: NIOSH Manual of Analytical Methods 4th edition

6. Answer: A

   $$F = \frac{9}{5}C + 32$$

   $$65 = \frac{9}{5}C + 32$$

   $$(65 - 32)\frac{5}{9} = C$$

   $$18.3 = C$$

7. Answer: A

   Explanation: Disorders affecting the vestibular system can cause loss of balance, vertigo, and nausea or vomiting. Examples of these disorders include viral labyrinthitis and Meniere's Disease. *Source: Fundamentals of Industrial Hygiene 5th edition*

8. Answer: D

   Explanation: The formula used to calculate the airborne concentration of fibers with the fiber density calculation in the numerator:

   $$C_{asb} = \frac{(C_s - C_b)A_c}{1000 \ (A_f)(V_s)}$$

   Where:
   C_{asb} is the airborne concentration of fibers in fibers per ml (f/ml).
   C_s is the average number of fibers counted per graticule field in the sample cassette filter.
   C_b is the average number of fibers counted per graticule field in the blank cassette filter.
   V_s is the volume of sampled air in liters.
   A_f is the graticule field area – approximately 0.00785 mm^2.
   A_c is the effective collection area of the filter, approximately 385 mm^2 for a 25 mm diameter film.

   $$V_s = 450 \text{ minutes x 2 L/m} = 900 \text{ L}$$

   $$C_{asb} = \frac{(3 - 0.01 \ fibers)385mm^2}{1000\frac{mL}{L} \ (0.00785mm^2)(900 \ L)}$$

   C_{asb} = 0.16 f/mL and since mL and cc are equivalent 0.16 f/cc

9. Answer B

   Explanation: First, calculate the number of moles required for neutralization.

   $$NaOH + HCl \rightarrow NaCl + H_2O$$

   So, 1 mole HCl neutralized 1 mole NaOH. The number of moles of NaOH is equivalent to volume x normality (moles/liter).

   $$0.0125 \text{ L x 0.15 N} = 0.001875 \text{ moles}$$

   Since 1 mole NaOH = 40g (molecular weight), then

   $$\text{wt} = 0.001875 \text{ moles x } \frac{40g}{g \, mole} = 0.074g$$

10. **Answer: B**

    Explanation: Antisepsis. This is the description found on the National Institute of Health webpage.

11. **Answer: D**

    Explanation: Studies have shown that the Andersen six-stage sieve impactor has greater sensitivity than the surface air systems (SAS). They are able to recover a significantly higher number of viable spores of Penicillium chrysogenum than the SAS system. Other reports comparing the SAS to slit to agar systems showed the SAS to be 50 percent, and 40 percent less efficient for sampling airborne fungi.

12. **Answer: B**

    Explanation: The fungus lives in the environment, particularly in moist soil and in decomposing matter such as wood and leaves. *Blastomyces* mainly live in areas of the United States and Canada surrounding the Ohio and Mississippi River valleys and the Great Lakes. People can get blastomycosis after breathing in the microscopic fungal spores from the air. Although most people who breathe in the spores do not get sick, some of those who do may have flu-like symptoms, and the infection can sometimes become serious if it is not treated. *Center for Disease Control, Fungi webpage*

13. **Answer: B**

    Explanation:

Table: Variance

Employee	Acetone Exposure (x_i)	$(\bar{x} - x_i)$	$(\bar{x} - x_i)^2$
1	15.9	-5.5	30.3
2	20.6	-10.2	104.0
3	11.9	-1.5	2.3
4	4.1	6.3	39.7
5	2.5	7.9	62.4
6	7.5	2.9	8.4
7	12.3	-1.9	3.6
8	8.4	2.0	4.0
Total	83.2	0	254.7

Calculate the variance:

$$s^2 = \frac{1}{(n-1)} \sum_{i=1}^{n} (\bar{x} - x_i)^2$$

$$s^2 = \frac{1}{(8-1)} \sum_{i=1}^{8} (10.40 - x_i)^2$$

$$s^2 = \frac{254.7}{7}$$

$$s^2 = 36.4 \ ppm^2$$

If you are using the TI 30X IIS, use the following calculation keystrokes:

Step 1 – Set to STAT Mode using the second function of DATA key

Step 2 – Select 1-VAR and Enter key

Step 3 – Press DATA key

Step 4 – Enter Data (X_1, down arrow key, FRQ, down arrow key; X_2, down arrow key, FRQ, down arrow key; … X_n, down arrow key, FRQ, down arrow key)

Step 5 – Press STATVAR key

Step 6 – Use arrow keys and select Sx

Step 7 – Square the value
Source: Industrial-Occupational Hygiene Calculations: A Professional Reference

14. Answer: C
   Explanation: Median - The exposure measurement that divides a set of measurements into two equal parts, with half less than and half greater than this value. *Source: Industrial-Occupational Hygiene Calculations: A Professional Reference*

15. Answer: C
   Explanation: Relative risk measures the association between exposure to a particular factor and risk of a health outcome. The relative risk expresses the absolute risk of one group with a factor (e.g., males, hypertensive, cigarette smokers) compared to the absolute risk of another group without such a factor (e.g., females, normotensives, nonsmokers).

$$\text{Relative Risk} = \frac{\text{Incidence rate among exposed}}{\text{Incidence rate among nonexposed}}$$

$$\text{Relative Risk} = \frac{\frac{20}{1000}}{\frac{4}{1000}} = \frac{0.02}{0.004} = 5$$

Source: Epidemiology 5th Edition, Leon Gordis

16. Answer: A

   Explanation: Gravity chambers are simple low flow, low efficiency devices that allow for particle settling. Cyclones use directional force to expel particles from the air stream. ESPs use electrical charge to attract particles. *Source: Air Pollution Control Engineering, 2nd Edition*

17. Answer: D

   Explanation: There are three main ways to deal with pollutants: prevention, dispersion (e.g., raise emission stacks), and collection and disposal (e.g., filters). *Source: Industrial Hygiene Reference and Study Guide, 3rd edition*

18. Answer: A

   Explanation: $NO_X + VOC \rightarrow O_3$
   Source: US EPA

19. Answer: C

   Explanation:

$$CFM\ 2 = 9,000\ CFM + 2,000\ CFM = 11,000\ CFM$$

$$\frac{RPM\ 2}{RPM\ 1} = \frac{CFM\ 2}{CFM\ 1}$$

$$RPM\ 2 = RPM\ 1 \left(\frac{CFM\ 2}{CFM\ 1}\right) = 1,500\ x\ \frac{11,000\ CFM}{9,000\ CFM}$$

$$RPM\ 2 = 1,833\ RPM$$

$$\frac{P\ 2}{P\ 1} = \left(\frac{RPM\ 2}{RPM\ 1}\right)^2$$

$$P\ 2 = P1 \left(\frac{RPM\ 2}{RPM\ 1}\right)^2$$

$$P\ 2 = 1.0 \left(\frac{1,833\ RPM}{1,500\ RPM}\right)^2$$

$$P\ 2 = 1.5\ inches\ wg$$

$$\frac{BHP\ 2}{BHP\ 1} = \left(\frac{RPM\ 2}{RPM\ 1}\right)^3$$

$$BHP\ 2 = BHP\ 1 \left(\frac{RPM\ 2}{RPM\ 1}\right)^3$$

$$BHP\ 2 = 5\ BHP \left(\frac{1,833\ RPM}{1,500\ RPM}\right)^3$$

$$BHP\ 2 = 9.1\ BHP$$

20. Answer: D
    Explanation:

$$V = 4005\sqrt{VP}$$

$$VP = 3.8 \text{ inches } WG$$

Step 1: Solve for V

$$V = 4005\sqrt{3.8}$$

$$V = 7807 \text{ FPM}$$

21. Answer: A
    Explanation:

$$C = \left(\frac{G}{Q'} \times 10^6\right) + C_{supply}$$

$$G = 8 \text{ CFM}$$
$$Q' = 2,700 \text{ CFM}$$
$$C_{supply} = 40 \text{ PPM}$$

$$C = \left(\frac{8 \text{ CFM}}{2,700 \text{ CFM}} \times 10^6\right) + 40 \text{ PPM} m_{supply}$$

$$C = 3,003 \text{ PPM}$$

Source: Industrial-Occupational Hygiene Calculations: A Professional Reference

22. Answer: B
    Explanation: *Thoracic outlet* syndrome results from compression of the nerves and blood vessels between the clavicle and the first and second ribs at the brachial plexus. This limits blood flow to the arm resulting in numbness and weakness. *Raynaud's* is also known as white finger syndrome. *Frozen shoulder* is a restricted range of motion and use due to inactivity, injury, or arthritic condition. *Source: The Occupational Environment, Its Evaluation, Control, and Management. 3rd edition*

23. Answer: A
    Explanation: Risk factors for the lower back include posture, frequency or repetition, static work, handles or coupling, asymmetrical handling, and space confinement. *Source: The Occupational Environment, Its Evaluation, Control, and Management. 3rd edition*

24. Answer: D

Explanation:

$$RWL = LC \times HM \times VM \times DM \times AM \times FM \times CM$$

$$RWL(kg) = 23\left(\tfrac{25}{H}\right)(1-.003\,|\,V-75\,|)\left(.82 + \tfrac{4.5}{D}\right)\left(1-(0.0032 \times A)\right)(FM)(CM)$$

$$RWL(kg) = 23\left(\tfrac{25}{45}\right)(1-.003 \times 0)\left(.82 + \tfrac{4.5}{25}\right)\left(1-(0.0032 \times 0)\right)(1)(1)$$

$$RWL(kg) = 23 \times 0.555 \times 1 \times 1 \times 1 \times 1 \times 1$$

$$RWL(kg) = 12.77 \text{ kg}$$

25. Answer: A

Explanation: Hazard is defined as the property of a chemical, physical or biological agent to render harm. A hazard is the source of risk. *Sources: (1) The Occupational Environment: Its Evaluation, Control and Management 3rd edition, Volume 1. (2) A Strategy for Assessing and Managing Occupational Exposures.*

26. Answer: C

Explanation:
Conversion from ppm to $\frac{mg}{m^3}$.

$$\frac{mg}{m^3} = \frac{(ppm)(\text{gram molecular weight of substance})}{24.45}$$

Where 24.45 = molar volume of air in liters at NTP conditions (25°C and 760 torr) and Molecular Weight $= \frac{g}{mol}$

$$\frac{mg}{m^3} = \frac{(ppm)(gram\ molecular\ weight\ of\ substance)}{24.45}$$

$$\frac{mg}{m^3} = \frac{(10ppm)(84.9\,\frac{g}{mol})}{24.45}$$

$$\frac{mg}{m^3} = 34.7$$

Source: TLVs and BEIS Based on the Documentation of the Threshold Limit Values for Chemical Substances and Physical Agents & Biological Exposure Indices

27. Answer: D
    Explanation:
    Step 1: Solve for d

$$d = \frac{0.61\lambda}{\eta sin\alpha}$$

$$d = \frac{0.61 \ x \ 450nm}{1.33 \ x \ 0.97}$$

d = 213 nm or 0.213 μm

28. Answer: A
    Explanation: According to the cross-functional program support relationship analysis developed by D. Polzo, the EHS tools are communicating, remediating, measuring, forecasting, training, investigation, interpretation, and guidance. *Source: The Occupational Environment: It's Evaluation, Control, and Management, 3rd Edition*

29. Answer: B
    Explanation: All of the answers are plausible; however, the ability to mobilize financial, human and other resources toward achieving organizational goals and vision is the most accepted description of modern leadership. *Source: The Occupational Environment: It's Evaluation, Control, and Management, 3rd Edition*

30. Answer: D
    Explanation:
    Step 1: Solve for percent error

$$\% \ error = \frac{(EV - TV)}{TV}$$

$$EV = 25 \ ppm$$
$$TV = 20 \ ppm$$

$$\% \ error = \frac{(25 \ ppm - 20 \ ppm)}{20 \ ppm}$$

$$\% \ error = 0.25 \ x \ 100$$

$$\% \ error = 25\%$$

31. Answer: B
    The noise exposure sampling results are presented in the table below.

Average dBA	90	92	86	84
C_i	2	1	3	2

Explanation:

Step 1: Calculate T_i for all levels listed in above table

$$T_i = \frac{8}{\left(2^{\left(\frac{L-90}{5}\right)}\right)} \, hours$$

$$T_i = \frac{8}{\left(2^{\left(\frac{90-90}{5}\right)}\right)} \, hours$$

$$T_i = \frac{8}{1}$$

$$T_i = 8.0 \, hours$$

$$T_i = \frac{8}{\left(2^{\left(\frac{92-90}{5}\right)}\right)} \, hours$$

$$T_i = \frac{8}{1.3}$$

$$T_i = 6.2 \, hours$$

$$T_i = \frac{8}{\left(2^{\left(\frac{86-90}{5}\right)}\right)} \, hours$$

$$T_i = \frac{8}{0.57}$$

$$T_i = 14 \, hours$$

$$T_i = \frac{8}{\left(2^{\left(\frac{84-90}{5}\right)}\right)} \, hours$$

$$T_i = \frac{8}{0.44}$$

$$T_i = 18.2 \, hours$$

Step 2: Calculate the Percent Dose

$$\%D = 100 \left[\frac{C_1}{T_1} + \frac{C_2}{T_2} + \cdots + \frac{C_i}{T_i}\right]$$

$$\%D = 100 \left[\frac{2}{8} + \frac{1}{6.2} + \frac{3}{14} + \frac{2}{18.2}\right]$$

$$\%D = 73.5 \, dB$$

Source: Source: Industrial-Occupational Hygiene Calculations: A Professional Reference

32. Answer: B
    Explanation:

$$TWA = 16.61 \, log\left(\frac{\%D}{100}\right) + 90 \, dBA$$

Step 1: Solve for TWA

$$TWA = 16.61 \, log\left(\frac{150}{100}\right) + 90 \, dBA$$

$$TWA = 93 \, dBA$$

Occupational Safety Calculations: A Professional Reference, 2nd Edition

33. Answer: C
    Explanation: By controlling at the source, the use of hearing protection devices may be eliminated. If effective, audiometric testing and other actions may be reduced. *Source: Noise and Hearing Conservation Manual, 4th Edition*

34. Answer: D
    Explanation: Z87.1 – 1989: American National Standard Practice for Occupational and Educational Eye and Face Protection. *Source: Industrial Hygiene Reference and Study Guide, 3rd edition*

35. Answer: D
    Explanation: ANSI Z89.1-2009 has the following hard hat classifications. Class G hard hats are for electrical use with low voltages (2,200 volts). Class E hard hats can be used with high voltages (22,000 volts). Class C hard hats conduct electricity and provide no electrical protection. *Source: American National Standards Institute (ANSI) Z89.12009*

36. Answer: C
    Explanation: Workplace temperature is the least likely to affect cartridge life of respirator chemical cartridges. All of the above have an effect on the service life of a cartridge with relative humidity having a major effect. A safety factor of 2 is recommended for RH above 65%, and experimental testing is recommended at levels of 85% or more. Increased temperature without an increase in RH may loosen attractive forces for the media to the contaminant. Another important factor is the volume of activated carbon in the cartridge. *OHSA.gov/SLTC/respiratory*

37. Answer: D
    Explanation: Ionization is the process of removing the electron, creating an ion pair. Photon mitigation and neutronization are non-related words. *Source: Industrial Hygiene Reference and Study Guide, 3rd edition*

38. Answer: B
   Explanation: Although no longer used as a glaze for Fiesta-Ware, Uranium was a popular orange glaze. Gamma and beta emissions can be detected from ceramics with this glaze. *Source: The Occupational Environment: Its Evaluation, Control and Management, 3rd Edition*

39. Answer: B
   Explanation: The gamma-ray constant equation can be used to estimate exposure.

$$D = \frac{\Gamma A}{d^2}$$

D = dose rate
A = activity
$d = d^2$

Step 1: Solve for D

$$D = \frac{\left(2.60 \frac{R - cm^2}{mCi - hr}\right)(0.003\ mCi)}{\left(20\ feet\left(\frac{30.48\ cm}{ft}\right)\right)^2}$$

$$D = 21.0 x 10^{-9} \frac{R}{hr}$$

$$D = 21.0x\ 10^{-3} \frac{\mu rem}{hr}$$

Step 2: Solve for Total Dose

$$Total\ dose = dose\ rate\ x\ time$$

$$Total\ dose = 21.0\ x\ 10^{-3} \frac{\mu rem}{hr}\ x\ 3\ hours$$

$$Total\ dose = 0.063\ \mu rem$$
Source: None provided

40. Answer: A
   Explanation: The penetration depth of UV into tissue is dependent on the wavelength, tissue thickness, and pigmentation (melanin). Wavelengths less than 300 nm are primarily absorbed in the epidermis, while wavelengths longer than 297 nm penetrate into the dermis. Erythema is reddening of the skin, and photosensitization is an abnormal skin reaction to UV in the presence of a chemical. Penetration is greater in fair skin than dark. *Source: Applications and Computational Elements of Industrial Hygiene, Stern and Mansdorf*

41. Answer: D

    Explanation: The main UV source is the sun. Global UV radiation has two components: the sun's beam and sky radiation. Sky radiation is diffuse and caused by scattering in the atmosphere. Global UV-A is a stable component of global radiation. Solar UV-B wavelengths less than about 295 nm are attenuated by stratospheric ozone, although wavelengths as low as 286 nm have been detected at the earth's surface. *Source: The Occupational Environment: Its Evaluation, Control, and Management 3rd Edition Volume 2*

42. Answer: C

    Explanation: Long wavelength to short wavelength: ELF → RF → Microwave → IR → Visible → UV. *Source: Industrial Hygiene Reference and Study Guide*

43. Answer: A

    Explanation: Conduction is the transfer of heat between two objects from the hotter to the colder object. Convection is the transfer of heat by air movement. Radiant heat is the transfer of heat using electromagnetic radiation, such as molten metal or the sun making the skin warm. *Source: Applications and Computational Elements of Industrial Hygiene, Stern and Mansdorf*

44. Answer: D

$$C = 7.0 \, V_{air}^{0.6}(t_{air} - t_{skin})$$

    Where:
    C = Convective heat exchange, kcal/hour
    V_{air} = Air velocity, meters per second
    t_{air} = Air temperature, °C
    t_{skin} = Mean weighted skin temperature (often assumed to be 35°C)

    Explanation: One potential source of heat load to the body is heat exchange between the air and skin of a worker. It is a function of air temperature, mean skin temperature, and wind speed.

$$C = 7.0 \, V_{air}^{0.6}(t_{air} - t_{skin})$$

$$C = 7.0 \, (5.8 \frac{m}{sec})^{0.6}(40°C - 35°C)$$

$$C = 100.5 \frac{kcal}{hr}$$

    Source: Applications and Computational Elements of Industrial Hygiene

45. Answer: B

    Explanation: Overexposure to lead may damage bone marrow. Carbon dioxide is relatively non-toxic, TDI is a sensitizer and beryllium exposure may result in lung disease.

46. Answer: B

    Explanation: CO is a chemical asphyxiant that reduces the blood's ability to transport oxygen.

47. Answer: A

    Explanation: Chemical oxidation involving a valence change from ferrous to ferric state creates the brownish-black pigment, methemoglobin.

48. Answer: A

    Explanation: Sulfur containing odorants include:

    tert-Butyl thiol (TBM), the main ingredient in many gas odorant blends.

    Tetrahydrothiophene (THT), used as an odorant for natural gas, usually in mixtures containing tert-butyl thiol.

    2-Propanethiol, commonly known as isopropyl mercaptan (IPM) is used as an odorant for natural gas, usually in mixtures containing tert-butyl thiol.

    Ethanethiol (EM), commonly known as ethyl mercaptan is used in liquefied petroleum gas (LPG), and resembles odor of leeks, onions, durian, or cooked cabbage.

    Dimethyl sulfide (DMS), a component of the smell produced from cooking of certain vegetables, notably maize, cabbage, beetroot, and sea foods. *Source: Pacific Natural Gas and Odorant Additive web page*

49. Answer: A

    Explanation: Infectious diseases caused by bacteria and viruses (e.g., flu, measles, chicken pox and tuberculosis) may be readily spread indoors. Most infectious diseases pass from person to person through physical contact. Crowded conditions with poor air circulation can promote this spread. Under certain conditions, some bacteria and viruses thrive in buildings and circulate through HVAC systems. For example, Legionella Pneumophila, the bacterium causing Legionnaire's disease (a serious and sometimes fatal infection) and Pontiac Fever (a flu-like illness), is known to thrive in and be disseminated by large HVAC systems or their cooling tower water. It is likely that the warning properties of formaldehyde would prevent fatal exposures, and in an office environment, lethal levels of carbon dioxide or formaldehyde are unlikely. *Source: The Occupational Environment: Its Evaluation, Control, and Management, 3rd Edition*

50. Answer: A

    Explanation: Fluoride causes irritation of the eyes and respiratory tract; absorption of excessive amounts of fluoride over a long period results in increased radiographic density of bone. A mottled appearance and an altered form of the teeth are produced only when excessive amounts of fluoride are ingested during the period of tooth formation and calcification, which occurs during the first 8 years of life in humans. After calcification has been completed, fluoride does not have an adverse effect on the teeth. *Source: Proctor and Hughes' Chemical Hazards of the Workplace, 3rd Edition*

Self-Assessment Exam 3

1. The lab detects 20 µg of toluene on the collection media. The industrial hygienist sampled for one hour at 0.05 L/m. What is the airborne concentration based on this sample?

    A) 400 ppm
    B) $0.2 \ \mu g/m^3$
    C) $670 \ mg/m^3$
    D) $6.67 \ mg/m^3$

2. A pump and sample media are calibrated to 2 L/m in the office. The calibration conditions are 69°F and 28 inches of Hg. The field conditions are 100°F and 29.2 inches of Hg. The sample duration was 7 hours and 40 minutes. Calculate the calibration volume and the field volume.

    A) 920 L, 934 L
    B) 920 L, 920 L
    C) 920 L, 891 L
    D) 920 L, 938 L

3. When is it appropriate for a TLV-STEL or TLV-C to take precedence over the excursion limit?

    A) The specific substance is being monitored for less than 10 minutes.
    B) Toxicologic data for a specific substance is available.
    C) Toxicologic data for a specific substance is not available.
    D) The specific substance is being monitored for over an 8-hour time period.

4. Select the gas chromatographic detector that is the most appropriate for analyzing polychlorinated biphenyls (PCBs).

    A) Thermal conductivity.
    B) Flame ionization.
    C) Electron capture.
    D) Flame photometric.

5. Choose the statement that best describes Chromatography.

    A) A separation technique that is generally used for inorganic compounds. The separation allows the quantitation of several compounds in multiple analysis.
    B) A separation technique that is generally used for organic compounds. The separation allows the quantitation of several compounds in a single analysis.
    C) A technique used to analyze organic compounds
    D) A separation technique that quantifies several compounds in multiple analysis.

6. A solution of methyl ethyl ketone in water is to be analyzed. The absorbance-concentration graph produces a straight line. If the molar absorptivity is 0.33 L/g-cm, the path length is 1 cm, and the absorbance is 0.400 at 265 nm, determine the concentration of the methyl ethyl ketone.

   A) 1.3 mg/m^3
   B) 1.21 g/L
   C) 12 ppm
   D) 33 μg/L

7. Hydrogen gas is measured at 2.5%. Express this values in parts per million.

   A) 250 ppm
   B) 25,000 ppm
   C) 250,000 ppm
   D) 2.5 million

8. An air sample for toluene (C_7H_8) was obtained under the following field conditions. The ambient temperature was 35°F, and the barometric pressure was 740 mmHg. The sample duration was 400 minutes with a flow of 0.5 L/m. The lab analysis detected 600μg on the media. Calculate the actual concentration of toluene in the air.

   A) 298 ppm
   B) 23 ppm
   C) 0.90 ppm
   D) 0.75 ppm

9. Which bacteria produces a heat stable toxin that can survive being boiled for 25 minutes in addition to tolerating salty conditions?

   A) Clostridium botulinum.
   B) Clostridium perfringens.
   C) Staphylococcus aureus.
   D) Helicobacter pylori.

10. Workers in the lumber industry who mill Western Red Cedar may develop asthma as a result of this sensitizer, which is present in the wood's dust:

    A) Diazomethane.
    B) Formaldehyde.
    C) Placatic Acid.
    D) Colophony.

11. Choose the statement that best describes filtration decontamination.

   A) Heat at 250°F under pressure (15-18 psi) in an autoclave. Most widely used and convenient method of sterilization.
   B) Membrane filters are used to remove bacteria, yeast, and molds from biologic and pharmaceutical solutions.
   C) Boil (212°F for > 30 minutes) and pasteurization (161°F for 15 seconds, or 143°F for 30 minutes) kills vegetative cells but not bacterial spores. High temperatures cause denaturation of enzymes and kill organisms
   D) Sterilization of new, prepackaged medical devices (e.g., syringes and catheters) and in bulk package sterilization in the delivery of food industries.

12. Two air samples are taken to measure a worker's exposure to tetrahydrofuran. One sample is collected for 260 minutes (T_1) and a concentration of 26.99ppm is found (this is C_1). A second sample is taken immediately after the first sample, for a period of 220 minutes (T_2) and a concentration (C_2) of 38.19ppm is measured. The SAE of the measurement of tetrahydrofuran is 0.10, and the PEL is 50ppm. The time-weighted average concentration (C_A) of both samples is 32.12ppm. Calculate the Lower Confidence Limit for Consecutive Samples.

   A) 0.60
   B) 1.87
   C) 2.61
   D) 5.98

13. Choose the statement that best describes the Coefficient of Variation.

   A) An important symmetric probability distribution characterized completely by two parameters: the mean and the standard deviation.
   B) An estimate of the parameter selected to represent the acceptability of an exposure profile.
   C) The sample standard deviation divided by the sample mean (or population parameters). When comparing variations between distributions with different means, coefficients of variation should be used. Sometimes expressed as a percentage.
   D) The distribution of a random variable with the property such that the logarithms of its values are normally distributed.

14. What is the incident rate of active cases of musculoskeletal injuries for a six-month period given the following?

- Population of workers at a construction company on March 30, 2017 = 200,000
- Number of new active cases of musculoskeletal injuries occurring between January 1 and June 30, 2017 = 88
- Number of active musculoskeletal injuries June 30, 2017 = 12

    A) 34 per 100,000 population
    B) 44 per 100,000 population
    C) 78 per 100,000 population
    D) 90 per 100,000 population
    E) 130 per 100,000 population

15. Concerning the Clean Air Act of 1970, what is the principal provision of section 109, National Ambient Air Quality Standards (NAAQS)?

A) Divides the country into regions. States must administer air quality in each such region, under federal supervision.
B) Establishes the Standards of Performance for New Stationary Sources.
C) Establishes National Ambient Air Quality Standards.
D) Places control on motor vehicle emissions primarily in the hands of the federal government; sets motor vehicle and fuel composition standards.

16. What is the overall efficiency of three series particulate collectors with efficiencies 75, 80, and 90%?

    A) 99.5%
    B) 95%
    C) 90%
    D) 80%

17. The diagram illustrates what type of plume?

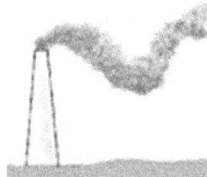

    A) Fanning.
    B) Fumigating.
    C) Looping.
    D) Coning.

18. An exhaust fan was selected for a particular industrial process to exhaust 40,000 CFM against a system static pressure of 4.0 inches WG when operating at 1,600 RPM and developing 20 BHP. Upon installation, it was discovered that the fan was actually exhausting 50,000 CFM. Use the fan law(s) to calculate the new operating speed for the fan to reduce exhaust volume to 40,000 CFM, as specified by the design selection.

   A)   900 RPM
   B)   1280 RPM
   C)   1440 RPM
   D)   1520 RPM

19. The laboratory hood operation plan requires the average face velocity to be between 90 and 110 FPM. With the sash open on the hood (18 inches) and no bypass feature, the average face velocity is 190 FPM. What height should the sash be set to in order to have a face velocity of 100 FPM?

   A)   8 inches
   B)   31.1 inches
   C)   34.2 inches
   D)   36 inches

20. Exhaust hoods capture contaminants and during the process converts duct static pressure to velocity pressure and hood entry losses. A hood static pressure is measured 6 duct diameters downstream from the hood. SP = -1.1 inches WG and VP = 1.3 inches WG. The hood is round and flanged. Calculate the hood entry loss.

   A)   0.64 inches WG
   B)   0.54 inches WG
   C)   0.49 inches WG
   D)   0.20 inches WG

21. NIOSH draws a distinction between ergonomics and work-related musculoskeletal disorders (WMSDs). Select the best description of WMSDs.

   A)   Injuries that involve the physiological and psychological stressors.
   B)   Injuries that include the nerves, tendons and supporting structures.
   C)   Disorders that effect the general well-being.
   D)   Hand-arm vibration syndrome.

22. Which of the following is not a factor in the NIOSH Work Practices Guide?

   A)   The horizontal distance of the load from the center of a line connecting the ankles at the beginning of the lift/lower.
   B)   The vertical distance the load travels.
   C)   The frequency of the lift/lower.
   D)   The weight of the worker.

23. The application of ergonomics emphasizes:

    A)   Selecting and training individuals to fit different jobs.
    B)   Designing jobs and tasks to fit people.
    C)   Decreasing worker complaint.
    D)   Meeting OSHA standards.

24. What is the appropriate method when sampling for chromic acid and chromates?

    A)   NIOSH 5500.
    B)   NIOSH 6890.
    C)   NIOSH 6500.
    D)   NIOSH 7600.

25. The lab reports 2 mg/m^3. Company protocol requires you to convert 2 milligrams per cubic meter of Tetrachloroethylene to parts per million. Reference information: Tetrachloroethylene: C_2Cl_4 Atomic Mass: C = 12 & Cl = 35.5

    A)   0.295
    B)   1.78
    C)   3.29
    D)   11.77

26. Calculate the weekly exposure reduction factor for a worker who works 8-hour shifts, seven days a week.

    A)   0.24
    B)   0.44
    C)   0.63
    D)   0.76

27. According to a company's safety professional, the following estimated errors are present in a sampling system.

    - Flow rate measurement ± 11%
    - Sampling time ± 2.8%
    - Collection efficiency ± 3.9%
    - Sample recovery ± 8.7%
    - Sample analysis ± 17%

    Calculate the cumulative error for the sampling system.

    A)   10.1%
    B)   22.6%
    C)   34.5%
    D)   40.3%

28. ISO 9000 is a consensus standard related to:

    A) Safety and Health Management.
    B) Environmental Auditing.
    C) Quality Management.
    D) International labor relations

29. An industrial hygienist uses an octave band analyzer to measure noise generated by a machine. Calculate the total sound intensity level on the A-scale for the following readings: 88 dB at 500 Hz, 94 dB at 1,000 Hz, 96 dB at 2,000 Hz.

    A) 90 dBA
    B) 99 dBA
    C) 103 dBA
    D) 109 dBA

30. What is the upper band-edge frequency of a one-third octave band whose lower band-edge frequency is 180 Hz?

    A) 90 Hz
    B) 136 Hz
    C) 169 Hz
    D) 227 Hz

31. A common type of frequency analysis uses an Octave Band Analyzer (OBA). This type of frequency analysis allows the user to measure frequencies (e.g., is equipped with band-pass filters). The width of the band is called an octave. An octave is where the upper frequency of the band is _____ the lower frequency of the band.

    A) Twice.
    B) Three times.
    C) Five times.
    D) Ten times.

32. ANSI Z 89.1 addresses protective headwear for industrial workers. The headwear is tested for penetration resistance, flammability and _____.

    A) Chemical resistance.
    B) Radiant heat transfer.
    C) Electrical hazards.
    D) Resistance to UV degradation.

33. Seamless rubber chemical gloves are used when employees work with paint remover (strong organic solvent). How would the employee's hands likely be first exposed to the solvent if the gloves are worn?

    A) The solvent could penetrate the glove.
    B) The solvent could degrade the glove.
    C) The solvent could permeate the glove.
    D) The solvent could corrode the glove.

34. The Occupational Safety and Health Administration (OSHA) defines an IDLH value in their hazardous waste operations and emergency response regulation as follows:

    An atmospheric concentration of any toxic, corrosive or asphyxiant substance that poses an immediate threat to life or would cause irreversible or delayed adverse health effects or would interfere with an individual's ability to escape from a dangerous atmosphere. [29 CFR* 1910.120]

    In the OSHA regulation on permit-required confined spaces, an IDLH condition is defined as follows:

    Any condition that poses an immediate or delayed threat to life or that would cause irreversible adverse health effects or that would interfere with an individual's ability to escape unaided from a permit space. **Note**: *Some materials--hydrogen fluoride gas and cadmium vapor, for example--may produce immediate transient effects that, even if severe, may pass without medical attention, but are followed by sudden, possibly fatal collapse 12-72 hours after exposure. The victim "feels normal" from recovery from transient effects until collapse. Such materials in hazardous quantities are considered to be "immediately dangerous to life or health."*

    ANSI considers confined space IDLH if the oxygen concentration is less than:

    A) 10.5%
    B) 15.8%
    C) 19.5%
    D) 20.9%

35. The measured radiation at 2 feet from the source is 100 mR/hr; assuming point source geometry, what is the source strength at 15 feet?

    A) 400 mR/hr
    B) 1.78 R/hr
    C) 40 R/hr
    D) 1.78 mR/hr

36. Readings are taken with a Geiger-Mueller tube 10 feet from the radiation source. The readings include the following: March 1: 60 mCi; March 8: 45 mCi; and March 16: 30 mCi.

   What is the measured activity level on April 3?

   A) 5.9 mCi
   B) 9.1 mCi
   C) 13 mCi
   D) 23.8 mCi

37. In regard to the shielding equation shown below, what if μ is larger than the shielding material for the photon energy of interest?

$$I = I_0 B e^{-\mu x}$$

   A) A material should have undermined shielding properties.
   B) No more effective than if μ were smaller.
   C) A more effective shield.
   D) A less effective shield.

38. What are the two general types of lasers?

   A) Steady beam laser and high frequency laser.
   B) High frequency laser and low frequency laser.
   C) Low frequency laser and pulsed laser.
   D) Steady beam laser and pulsed laser.

39. Chronic corneal exposure to subthreshold doses of IR may lead to "dry eye." How is "dry eye" characterized?

   A) Photosensitivity.
   B) Conjunctivitis.
   C) Conjunctivitis and Decreased Lacrimation.
   D) Decreased Lacrimation, Photosensitivity and Conjunctivitis.

40. Example Laser Problem: What is the minimal Optical Density (OD) required of protective eyewear?

   Given:
   ML (Measured Level) = 128 mW/cm^2
   EL (Exposure Limit) = 0.0190 mW/cm^2

   A) 3.83
   B) 4.78
   C) 9.50
   D) 12.78

41. Normal body functioning is maintained, in part, by the body's ability to maintain a relatively constant core temperature. Heat is generated internally by metabolic activity. Which part of the central nervous system is responsible for thermoregulation in humans?

    A) Heat cramps
    B) Medulla oblongata
    C) Cerebellum
    D) Hypothalamus

42. Using the equation below, calculate the heat stress index for a worker that has a required evaporation of 40 kcal/hour and a maximal evaporation of 100 kcal/hour. Use the evaluation of heat stress index table to determine the physiologic and hygienic implications of 8-hour exposures to heat stress index.

    A) -20, Mild cold strain
    B) 0, No thermal strain
    C) +40, Severe heat strain
    D) +70, Very severe heat strain

$$HSI = \left(\frac{E_{req}}{E_{max}}\right) x \, 100$$

Evaluation of Heat Stress Index

Heat Stress Index	Physiologic and Hygienic Implications of 8-hour Exposures to Heat Stress Index
+100	• Maximum strain tolerated by fit, acclimatized young workers.
+70	• Very severe heat strain. • Only a small percentage of the population may be expected to qualify for this work. Personnel should be selected (a) by medical examination and (b) by trial on the job (after acclimatization). • Special measures are needed to assure adequate water and salt intake. • Amelioration of work conditions by any feasible means is highly desirable and may be expected to decrease the health hazard, while increasing efficiency on the job. • Slight "indisposition", which in most jobs would be insufficient to affect performance, may render workers unfit for this exposure.
+40	• Severe heat strain involving a threat to health unless workers are physically fit. • Break periods are required for workers not previously acclimatized. • Some decrement in performance of physical work is to be expected. • Medical selection of personnel is desirable because these conditions are unsuitable for those with cardiovascular or respiratory impairments or with chronic dermatitis. • These working conditions are also unsuitable for activities requiring sustained mental effort.
+10	• Mild to moderate heat strain. • For a job that involves higher intellectual function, dexterity, or alertness, subtle to substantial decrements in performance are expected. • In the performance of heavy physical work, little decrement is expected unless the ability of individuals to perform such work under marginal stress would be expected to be detrimental.
0	• No thermal strain.
-20	• Mild cold strain. • This condition frequently exists in areas where recovery from exposures to heat occurs.

43. Which of the following engineering controls would be the best solution to provide protection against heat stress in an indoor manufacturing environment?

    A) Large fans to increase air movement
    B) Worker Rotation program to limit worker exposure to heat stress
    C) Dilution ventilation that pulls make up air from the outside
    D) Providing employees with cooling vests

44. The mechanism of action for both organophosphate and carbamate insecticides is:

    A) Inhibition of acetylcholinesterase activity.
    B) Inhibition of acetylcholine activity.
    C) Promotion of acetylcholinesterase activity.
    D) Inhibition of beta-naphthalene activity.

45. Occupational exposure is most likely to occur via:

    A) Inhalation.
    B) Dermal absorption.
    C) Ingestion.
    D) Oral Uptake.

46. When evaluating a dose response curve (response on article axis, dose on horizontal axis) the distance from the y-axis to the beginning of the curve is known as:

    A) The LD 50.
    B) The LC 50.
    C) The threshold distances.
    D) The lethal point.

47. Pulp-paper manufacturing may utilize the Kraft process. The Kraft process utilizes a mixture of sodium hydroxide and sodium sulfide (white liquor) that breaks links between lignin and cellulose. Exposures occur when workers open the bottom of the digester and dump the contents. What exposures can be anticipated during this activity?

    A) Hydrogen chloride, calcium chloride.
    B) Hydrogen sulfide, sulfur dioxide.
    C) Hydrogen cyanide, sodium cyanide.
    D) Hydrogen, chlorine.

48. A(n) _____ is a written program which sets forth procedures, equipment, personal protective equipment, and work practices that are capable of protecting employees from the health hazards presented by hazardous chemicals used in the particular workplace.

    A) Industrial Hygiene Plan.
    B) Chemical Hygiene Plan.
    C) Lab Safety Plan.
    D) RCRA Plan.

49. Choose the statement that correctly describes the distribution of absorbed lead in the body.

    A) Blood → Bone → Soft Tissue
    B) Soft Tissue → Bone → Blood
    C) Blood → Soft Tissue → Bone
    D) Bone → Soft Tissue → Blood

50. Which is the best definition of hazard?

    A) A condition, set of circumstances, or inherent property that can cause injury, illness, or death.
    B) An event in which a work-related injury or illness or fatality occurred or could have occurred.
    C) A set of interrelated elements that establish and support occupational safety and health objectives.
    D) An estimate of the combination of the likelihood of an occurrence of a hazardous event or exposure, and the severity of the injury.

Self-Assessment Exam 3 Answers

1. Answer: D
   Explanation:
   Calculate the volume of air sampled:

   $$\text{Flow Rate x Time} = \text{Volume}$$

   $$0.05 \text{ L/m x } 60 \text{ minutes} = 3 \text{ L}$$

   $$3 \text{ L x } 1 \text{ m}^3/1000 \text{ L} = 0.003 \text{ m}^3$$

   Convert µg to mg:

   $$20 \text{ µg x } 1 \text{ mg}/1000 \text{ µg} = 0.02 \text{ mg}$$

   Calculate the concentration:

   $$\frac{0.02 \, mg}{0.003 m^3} = 6.67 \frac{mg}{m^3}$$

2. Answer: A
   Explanation:
   Use this expression:

   $$V_{field} = V_{cal}\left(\frac{T_{field}}{T_{cal}}\right)\left(\frac{P_{cal}}{P_{field}}\right)$$

   Convert conditions to absolute conditions:

   $$T_{cal} = 69 + 460 = 529° \text{ R}$$

   $$T_{field} = 100 + 460 = 560° \text{ R}$$

   $$P_{cal} = 28 \text{ inches Hg } \left(\frac{25.4 \, mm}{1 \, inch}\right) = 711.2 \text{ mmHg}$$

   $$P_{cal} = 29.2 \text{ inches Hg } \left(\frac{25.4 \, mm}{1 \, inch}\right) = 741.7 \text{ mmHg}$$

   Calculate the volume for calibration conditions:

   $$\text{FR x T} = V_{cal}$$

   $$2 \text{ L/m x } 460 \text{ m} = 920 \text{ L}$$

   Insert knowns and solve for V_{field}:

   $$V_{field} = V_{cal}\left(\frac{T_{field}}{T_{cal}}\right)\left(\frac{P_{cal}}{P_{field}}\right)$$

$$V_{field} = 920L_{cal}\left(\frac{560_{field}}{529_{cal}}\right)\left(\frac{711.2_{cal}}{741.7_{field}}\right)$$

$$V_{field} = 933.9 \text{ L or } 934 \text{ L}$$

Source: Fundamentals of Industrial Hygiene 6th ed. NSC

3. Answer: B

Explanation: If exposure excursions are maintained within the recommended limits, the geometric standard deviation of the concentration measurements will be near 2.0, and the goal of the recommendations will be accomplished. It is recognized that the geometric standard deviations of some common workplace exposures may exceed 2.0. If such distributions are known and workers are not at increased risk of adverse health effects, recommended excursion limits should be modified based upon workplace-specific data. When the toxicologic data for a specific substance is available to establish a TLV-STEL or a TLV-C, these values take precedence over the excursion limit. *Source: TLVs and BEIs Based on Documentation of the Threshold Limit Values for Chemical Substances and Physical Agents & Biological Exposure Indices*

4. Answer: B

Explanation: The Flame Ionizing Detector (FID) is simple and measures total mass rather than concentration. It responds with "cleaner" PCB profiles. (The most common errors in this process are insufficient sample extraction and inappropriate sample clean-up.) *Source: Buck Scientific GC 3011 publication*

5. Answer: B

Explanation: Chromatography is a separation technique that is generally used for detection of organic compounds. The separation allows the quantitation of several compounds in a single analysis. The three types of chromatography are Gas Chromatography (GC), High Performance Liquid Chromatography (HPLC), and Ion Chromatography (IC). *Sources: (1) The Occupational Environment: Its Evaluation, Control and Management, 3rd edition. (2) Applications and Computational Elements of Industrial Hygiene*

6. Answer: B

$$\log\frac{I_0}{I} = abc$$

$$\log\frac{I_0}{I} = abc = \text{absorbance}$$
$$\text{absorbance} = 0.400$$
$$a = 0.33 \text{ L/g-cm}$$
$$b = 1 \text{ cm}$$
$$c = ?$$

Step 1: Solve for the concentration-c

$$0.400 = 0.33 \text{ L/g-cm}(1 \text{ cm})(c)$$

$$\frac{0.400}{\left(0.33\frac{L}{g-cm}\right)(1 \text{ cm})} = c$$

$$1.21 \text{ g/L} = c$$

7. Fill in the chart.

Answer: B

Explanation: 1% equals 10,000 parts per million, 2.5 x 10,000 = 25,000

8. Answer: D

   Explanation:

   Step 1: Calculate the volume of air collected

   $$402 \text{ min x } \frac{0.5 \text{ L}}{min} x \frac{1 m^3}{1000L} = 0.201 \text{ m}^3$$

   Step 2: Calculate the exposure concentration

   $$\frac{600 \text{ ug}}{0.201 m^3} x \frac{1 \text{ mg}}{1000 \text{ ug}} = 2.98 \frac{mg}{mg^3}$$

   Step 3: Calculate the concentration in ppm under field conditions

   Use Ideal Gas Law to determine molar volume of field conditions

   $$\frac{P_1 V_1}{T_1} = \frac{P_2 V_2}{T_2}$$

   Note: All must be in absolute units

   $$35°F = 1.7°C = 274.7°K$$
   $$25°C = 298°K$$

   $$\frac{760 x 24.45}{298} = \frac{740 x V_2}{274.7}$$

   $$V_2 = 23.15 \text{ L}$$

   The molecular weight of $C_7H_8 = 92$

$$ppm = \frac{2.98\ mg/m^3 x\ 23.15}{92}$$

$$= 0.75\ ppm$$

9. Answer: C
   Explanation: Staphylococcus aureus produces a heat stable toxin that allows it to survive boiling for 25 minutes. It is also tolerant of salty environments.

10. Answer: C
    Explanation: Plicatic acid causes asthma in workers who are exposed to Western Red Cedar Wood dust. Occupational exposure to cedar and pine woods, and pine resin (colophony), can cause asthma and chronic lung disease. Prior studies suggest that plicatic and abietic acids are responsible for the asthmatic reactions that occur in cedarwood and colophony workers. *The Toxicity of Constituents of Cedar and Pine Woods to Pulmonary Epithelium. Journal of Allergy and Clinical Immunology*

11. Answer: B

Table: Physical Agent Decontamination Techniques and Process/Application

Technique	Process/Application
Steam	Heat at 250°F under pressure (15-18 psi) in an autoclave. Most widely used and convenient method of sterilization.
Wet Heat	Boil (212°F for > 30 minutes) and pasteurization (161°F for 15 seconds, or 143°F for 30 minutes) kills vegetative cells but not bacterial spores. High temperatures cause denaturation of enzymes and kill organisms.
Dry Heat	Open flames and Bacti-Cinerators (tm) (an electrical device that dry-heats at 1600°F) are used to heat sterilize inoculation loops. Hot air ovens (160-180°C for 2 hours) are used for anhydrous materials (e.g., greases and powders). Incinerators are used to destroy infectious waste.
Ionizing Radiation	Sterilization of new, prepackaged medical devices (e.g., syringes and catheters) and in bulk package sterilization in the delivery of food industries.
Ultraviolet (UV) Radiation	Inactivation of viruses, mycoplasma, bacteria, and fungi. Least effective and least perfected method of sterilization. Not practical as a disinfectant of liquids.
Filtration	Membrane filters are used to remove bacteria, yeast, and molds from biologic and pharmaceutical solutions. Common spore sizes: 0.22µm, 0.45µm, and 0.8µm

Source: The Occupational Environment: Its Evaluation, Control, and Management, 3rd edition

12. Answer: A

    Explanation:

    Calculate the Lower Confidence Limit for Consecutive Samples

    $$LCL = \frac{C_A}{PEL} - \frac{SAE\sqrt{T_1^2 C_1^2 + T_2^2 C_2^2 + \cdots + T_n^2 C_n^2}}{PEL(T_1 + T_2 + \cdots T_n)}$$

    $$LCL = \frac{32.12ppm}{50ppm} - \frac{0.10\sqrt{(26.99ppm)^2(260min)^2 + (38.19ppm)^2(220min)^2}}{50ppm(260min + 220min)}$$

    $$LCL = 0.5968$$

    Therefore, the exposure exceeds the PEL at the 95% confidence level. *Source: Industrial-Occupational Hygiene Calculations: A Professional Reference*

13. Answer: C

    Explanation:
    Coefficient of Variation: The sample standard deviation divided by the sample mean (or population parameters). When comparing variations between distributions with different means, coefficients of variation should be used. Sometimes expressed as a percentage. Abbreviated CV. *Source: Industrial-Occupational Hygiene Calculations: A Professional Reference*

14. Answer B

    Explanation: Calculate the incident rate:

    $$Incidence\ Rate = \frac{number\ of\ new\ cases\ of\ a\ disease\ in\ the\ time\ period}{population\ at\ risk\ of\ the\ disease\ in\ the\ time\ period}$$

    $$Incidence\ Rate = \frac{88}{200,000} = 0.00044\ x\ 100,000 = 44\ per\ 100,000\ population$$

    Source: Epidemiology 5th Edition, Leon Gordis

15. Answer: C
Explanation:

Sections of the Clean Air Act of 1970, as Amended in 1977 and 1990

Section	Title	Provisions
107	Air Quality Control Regions (AQCR)	Divides the country into regions. States must administer air quality in each such region, under federal supervision.
109	National Ambient Air Quality Standards (NAAQS)	Establishes National Ambient Air Quality Standards.
110	State Implementation Plans (SIP)	Requires states to prepare and enforce State Implementation Plans. Gives details on how it has to be accomplished.
111	New Source Performance Standards (NSPS)	Establishes the Standards of Performance for New Stationary Sources.
112 and 301-306	National Emission Standards for Hazardous Air Pollutants (NESHAP)	Establishes National Emission Standards for Hazardous Air Pollutants, also called air toxics.
160-169	Prevention of Significant Deterioration (PSD)	Lays out rules and regulations for regions with air cleaner than the NAAQS and for the protection of visibility, principally in the large national parks and wilderness areas.
171-192	Nonattainment areas	Gives detailed descriptions of what must be done in areas where NAAQS are not currently met.
202-235	Mobile sources	Places control on motor vehicle emissions mostly in the hands of the federal government; sets motor vehicle and fuel composition standards.
401-416	Acid deposition control	Establishes a federal acid deposition control program.
601-618	Stratospheric ozone protection	Establishes programs for protection of the stratospheric ozone layer.

Source: US EPA

16. Answer: A
    Explanation:

100% → [ ] --- 25% --- [ ] → (.2) (.25) = 5% -- [ ] .10 (.05) =
.005

75%   (.8)(.25) = 20%   (.9) (0.05) =
0.04

Source: U of U

17. Answer: C
    Explanation: Looping plumes occur when there are unstable conditions. *Industrial Hygiene Reference and Study Guide. 3rd Edition*

18. Answer: B
    Explanation:

$$\frac{CFM\ 1}{CFM\ 2} = \frac{RPM\ 1}{RPM\ 2}$$

$$\frac{50,000\ CFM}{40,000\ CFM} = \frac{1,600\ RPM}{RPM\ 2}$$

$$1.25\ x\ RPM\ 2 = 1,600\ RPM$$

$$RPM\ 2 = 1,280\ RPM$$

19. Answer: C
    Explanation: It assumed that the airflow remains constant. The width of the hood is also constant. Set up an equality and solve for the height.

$$18\ inches\ x\ 190\ FPM = Height_2 x\ 100\ FPM$$

$$\frac{18\ inches\ x\ 190\ FPM}{100\ FPM} = Height_2$$

$Height_2$ = 34.2 inches or 2.85 feet

20. Answer: A
    Explanation:
    Step 1: Obtain the loss factor from the formula sheet
    $$f_h = 0.49$$

    Step 2: Calculate the hood entry loss
    $$h_e = f_h \, x \, VP_d$$

    $$h_e = 0.49 \; x \; 1.3$$

    h_e = 0.64 inches WG
    Source: IH Workbook, 6th edition, Burton

21. Answer: B
    Explanation: WMSDs include a group of conditions that involve the nerves, tendons, and supporting structures, including the intervertebral discs. A wide range of disorders that can be mild, periodic, severe, or chronic and debilitating. *Source: The Occupational Environment, Its Evaluation, Control, and Management. 3rd edition*

22. Answer: D
    Explanation: The weight of the worker is not a factor in the NIOSH Work Practices Guide. The following are in the NIOSH Work Practices Guide: the horizontal distance of the load from the center of a line connecting the ankles at the beginning of the lift/lower; the vertical location of the load from the floor at the beginning of the lift/lower; the vertical distance that the load travels; and the frequency of the lift/lower. *Source: CDC/NIOSH*

23. Answer: B
    Explanation: Ergonomics is the study of human characteristics for the appropriate design of the living and work environment. Ergonomic researchers strive to learn about human characteristics (capabilities, limitations, motivations, and desires) so that this knowledge can be used to adapt a human-made environment to the people involved. This knowledge may affect complex technical systems or work tasks, equipment, and workstations, or the tools and utensils used at work, at home, or during leisure times. Hence, ergonomics is human-centered, transdisciplinary, and application-oriented. *Source: Fundamentals of Industrial Hygiene 5th Edition*

24. Answer: D
    Explanation: According to the NIOSH Manual of Analytical Methods, the appropriate method when sampling for Chromic acid and chromates is NIOSH 7600. The OSHA analytical method that is currently preferred is OSHA ID 215. The OSHA ID 215 method uses an Ion Chromatograph equipped with a UV-Vis detector. *Sources: (1) NIOSH Manual of Analytical Methods 4th edition. (2) OSHA Technical Center.*

25. Answer: A
   Explanation:
   Conversion from $\frac{mg}{m^3}$ to ppm.

   $$ppm = \frac{(\frac{mg}{m^3})(24.45)}{(\text{gram molecular weight of substance})}$$

   Where, 24.45 = molar volume of air in liters at NTP conditions (25°C and 760 torr) and Molecular Weight = $\frac{g}{mol}$

   $$ppm = \frac{(\frac{mg}{m^3})(24.45)}{(\text{gram molecular weight of substance})}$$

   $$ppm = \frac{(2\frac{mg}{m^3})(24.45)}{(165.8\frac{g}{mol})}$$

   $$ppm = 0.295$$

   Source: TLVs and BEIS Based on the Documentation of the Threshold Limit Values for Chemical Substances and Physical Agents and Biological Exposure Indices

26. Answer: C
   Explanation: Using the Brief and Scala reduction for extended workweeks, if the shift is 8-hours per day, calculate the reduction factor.

   $$RF = \frac{40}{h_w} x \frac{168 - h_w}{128}$$

   $$RF = \frac{40}{56} x \frac{168 - 56}{128}$$

   $$RF = 0.71 \text{ x } 0.875$$

   $$RF = 0.625 \text{ or } 0.63$$

27. Answer: B
   o Flow rate measurement $\pm 11\%$
   o Sampling time $\pm 2.8\%$
   o Collection efficiency $\pm 3.9\%$
   o Sample recovery $\pm 8.7\%$

○ Sample analysis ± 17%

Step 1: Solve for the cumulative error

$$E_c = \sqrt{[(E_1)^2 + (E_2)^2 + (E_3)^2 + (E_4)^2 + (E_5)^2]}$$

$$E_c = sampling\ system\ cumulative\ error\ (\%)$$
$$E_i = error\ number\ i\ (\%)$$

$$E_1 = 11\%$$
$$E_2 = 2.8\%$$
$$E_3 = 3.9\%$$
$$E_4 = 8.7\%$$
$$E_5 = 17\%$$

$$E_c = \sqrt{[(11)^2 + (2.8)^2 + (3.9)^2 + (8.7)^2 + (17)^2]}$$

$$E_c = \sqrt{121 + 7.8 + 15.2 + 75.7 + 289}$$

$$E_c = \sqrt{508.7}$$

$$E_c = 22.6\%$$

28. Answer: C

    Explanation: International Organization for Standardization 9000 is a Quality Management consensus standard that requires a quality policy and a system that is adequate, documented, implemented and meets all specified requirements. ISO 1400 is a consensus standard for environmental management. It lists the basic elements of an effective management system as policy, objectives/standards, implementation of effective program, monitoring and measuring program effectiveness, correcting deficiencies, and review for continual improvement. *Source: Industrial Hygiene Reference and Study Guide, 3rd Edition*

29. Answer: B

    Explanation: The A-weighted sound level measurement is an appropriate assessment of overall noise hazard because it provides a rating of industrial broadband noises that indicates the injurious effects noise has on human hearing. A weighted-frequency scale is a series of correction factors that are applied to sound pressure levels on an energy basis as a function of frequency. The table below displays the corrections for the A-weighted network at each of the octave-band center.

Table: Octave-Band Correction Factors of the A-Weighted Network

Octave-Band Center Frequency (Hz)	A-Network Correction Factor (dB)
250	-8.6
500	-3.2
1,000	0
2,000	1.2
4,000	1.0

Step 1: Make the A-scale adjustments

$$88.0 - 8.6 = 85 dBA \text{ at } 250\ Hz$$

$$94.0 - 0.0 = 94\ dBA \text{ at } 1,000\ Hz$$

$$96.0 + 1.0 = 97\ dBA\ @\ 4,000\ Hz$$

Step 2: Calculate the total sound pressure level

$$L_{Pt} = 10log\left(\sum_{i=l}^{n} 10^{Lp_i/10}\right)$$

$$L_{Pt} = 10log\left(10^{\frac{79}{10}} + 10^{\frac{94}{10}} + 10^{\frac{97}{10}}\right)$$

$$L_{Pt} = 99\ dBA$$

Source: Fundamentals of Industrial Hygiene 5th Edition

30. Answer: D
Explanation:

$$f_2 = \sqrt[3]{2f_1}$$

Step 1: Solve for f_2

$$f_2 = \sqrt[3]{2}\,(180)$$

$$f_2 = 227\ Hz$$

Source: Industrial-Occupational Hygiene Calculations: A Professional Reference

31. Answer: A
Explanation: The width of the band is an octave. An octave is where the upper frequency of the band is twice the lower frequency of the band. *Source: Industrial Hygiene Reference and Study Guide, 3rd edition*

32. Answer: C
Head protection consists of two types: **Type I and Type II.**

Type I hard hats are only designed to protect workers from objects and blows that come from above and strike the top of a helmet.

Type II hard hats are designed to offer protection from lateral blows and objects, including from the front, back, side and top. Type II hard hats are also tested for off-center penetration resistance and chin strap retention.

Classes

Hard hats are also divided into classes that indicate how well they protect against electrical shock.
- *Class E (Electrical)* hard hats can withstand up to 20,000 volts of electricity.
- *Class G (General)* hard hats are able to withstand 2,200 volts of electricity.
- *Class C (Conductive)* hard hats offer no protection from electric shock.

There were three main changes to the ANSI/ISEA Z89.1-2014 standard issued on May 15, 2014:

- Under the section of *Accessories and Replacement Components,* there is further clarification that accessory or component manufacturers are required to prove that their components do not cause the helmets to fail. Helmet accessory or component suppliers must provide justification upon request that their product would not cause the helmet to fail the requirements of the Head Protection Standard.

- Additional language added under the *Instructions* and *Markings* section to help clarify that "useful service life" for helmets is not required by the Standard. It is up to helmet manufacturers if they want to include specific service life in terms of years. Manufacturers could elect to specify the number of years for their helmet's service life or elect to identify certain conditions that may affect a helmet's protection capability over time.

- The last section revised was the Higher Temperature section for users who work in hot environments. This section was updated to incorporate an optional preconditioning at a higher temperature of 140° F +/- 3.6° F (60° C +/- 2° C). Previously hot temperature preconditioning was conducted at 120° F +/- 3.6° F (48.8° C +/- 2° C) under the 2009 Standard. Helmets that meet the performance criteria after being preconditioned to these higher temperatures (140° F) will be designated with a HT marking.

33. Answer: C

    Explanation: Strong organic solvents will permeate most materials, including synthetic rubber. *Permeation* is the process by which chemical moves through a protective clothing material on a molecular basis. *Degradation* is the process of changing the chemical make-up of the material (e.g., material dissolves). *Penetration* is the direct flow of a chemical through closures, seams, pinholes, or other imperfections in the protective clothing material. *Source: OSHA Technical Manual & Fundamentals of Industrial Hygiene 5th Edition*

34. Answer: D

Explanation: ANSI Z88.27.3.3- Special considerations for confined spaces. Confined spaces continue to be the cause of numerous deaths and serious injuries. Therefore, any confined space containing less than 20.9% oxygen is to be considered IDLH, unless the source of the oxygen reduction is understood and controlled. *Source: OSHA.gov &American National Standards Institute*

35. Answer: D

Step 1: Use the inverse square law to solve for the strength (intensity) $\frac{I_1}{I_2} = \left[\frac{d_2}{d_1}\right]^2$

$$\frac{100 \; mr/Hr}{I_2} = \left[\frac{15 \; feet}{2 \; feet}\right]^2$$

$$I_2 = 100\frac{mr}{hr} \; x \left[\frac{2 \; feet}{15 \; feet}\right]^2$$

$$I_2 = 1.78 \text{ mR/hr}$$

36. Answer: C

Step 1: Calculate the half-life

Note: An examination of the data shows that at 15 days, the activity is ½ the initial activity level. The half-life is 15 days.

$$A_t = A_0\left(0.5^{\left(\frac{t}{T1/2}\right)}\right)$$

Step 2: Use the equation to determine the activity at time, t (April 3 = 33 days)

$$A_t = 60\left(0.5^{\left(\frac{33}{15}\right)}\right)$$

$$A_t = 13 \text{ mCi}$$

37. Answer: C

Explanation: This equation calculates the attenuation when a shield is placed between a detector and a point source of x or γ rays. The linear attenuation coefficient (μ) is strongly dependent on the shield composition and energy of the radiation. The shield becomes more effective as the interacting portion grows larger.
Source: Useful Equations for Radiation, Wright State University

38. Answer: D

Explanation: There are two general types of lasers. The first type of laser generates a continuous wave of light that is emitted as a steady beam. This type of laser has a peak power equal to the average power output, and the beam irradiance is constant with time. Continuous-wave (CW) lasers emit a "temporally constant power of laser light." The second type of laser is the pulsed laser. The pulsed laser has a mode of operation that consists of the emission of either a single pulse, or a series of laser pulses, with pulse periods ranging from a few picoseconds to seconds. Pulsed lasers may be normal pulse, Q-switched, or mode-locked. *Source: The Occupational Environment: Its Evaluation, Control and Management 3rd Ed., Volume 2*

39. Answer: B
    Explanation: IR produces thermal effects to the eye. The cornea is highly transparent to IR-A, has water absorption bands at 1.43 and 1.96 μm and becomes opaque to IR above 2.5μm. Chronic corneal exposure to subthreshold doses may lead to "dry eye," characterized by conjunctivitis and decreased lacrimation. *Source: The Occupational Environment: Its Evaluation, Control, and Management 3rd Edition Volume 2*

40. Answer: A
    Explanation:

$$O.D._{needed} = \log\left[\frac{ML}{EL}\right] = \log_{10}\left[\frac{128 \text{ mW/cm}^2}{0.0190 \text{ mW/cm}^2}\right] = \log_{10}[6737] = 3.83$$

Source: University of Utah Comprehensive Review of Industrial Hygiene

41. Answer: D
    Explanation: Through neural transmitters, the hypothalamus is able to sense temperature changes in the skin, muscle, stomach, etc., and signal either heat conserving or heat dissipating mechanisms. *Source: Applications and Computational Elements of Industrial Hygiene, Stern and Mansdorf*

42. Answer: C
    Explanation:

$$HSI = \left(\frac{E_{req}}{E_{max}}\right) x \ 100$$

$$HSI = \left(\frac{40 \text{ kcal/hour}}{100 \text{ kcal/hour}}\right) x \ 100$$

$$HSI = 40, \text{ Severe heat strain}$$

Source: Applications and Computational Elements of Industrial Hygiene

Evaluation of Heat Stress Index

Heat Stress Index	PHYSIOLOGIC AND HYGIENIC IMPLICATIONS OF 8-HOUR EXPOSURES TO HEAT STRESS INDEX
+100	• Maximum strain tolerated by fit, acclimatized young workers.
+70	• Very severe heat strain. • Only a small percentage of the population may be expected to qualify for this work. Personnel should be selected (a) by medical examination and (b) by trial on the job (after acclimatization). • Special measures are needed to assure adequate water and salt intake. • Amelioration of work conditions by any feasible means is highly desirable and may be expected to decrease the health hazard, while increasing efficiency on the job. • Slight "indisposition", which in most jobs would be insufficient to affect performance, may render workers unfit for this exposure.
+40	• Severe heat strain involving a threat to health unless workers are physically fit. • Break periods are required for workers not previously acclimatized. • Some decrement in performance of physical work is to be expected. • Medical selection of personnel is desirable because these conditions are unsuitable for those with cardiovascular or respiratory impairments or with chronic dermatitis. • These working conditions are also unsuitable for activities requiring sustained mental effort.
+10	• Mild to moderate heat strain. • For a job that involves higher intellectual function, dexterity, or alertness, subtle to substantial decrements in performance are expected. • In the performance of heavy physical work, little decrement is expected unless the ability of individuals to perform such work under marginal stress would be expected to be detrimental.
0	• No thermal strain.
-20	• Mild cold strain. • This condition frequently exists in areas where recovery from exposures to heat occurs.

$$HSI = \left(\frac{E_{req}}{E_{max}}\right) x\ 100$$

43. Answer: C

    Explanation: Dilution ventilation is the best solution because it uses cooler outside make up air to replace the hot air in the building. While using large fans is a viable option in some manufacturing environments, the fans do not address the temperature of the air. Using a worker rotation and providing cooling vests are administrative controls, which will not do anything to address the heat in the manufacturing environment.

44. Answer: A

    Explanation: Organophosphate and carbamate insecticides affect the autonomic nervous system by inhibiting acetylcholinesterase (an enzyme that breaks down the neurotransmitter acetylcholine).

45. Answer: B

    Explanation: Parathion readily penetrates skin. It also has a low vapor pressure that makes inhalation less likely.

46. Answer: C

    Explanation: The beginning of the curve is the threshold for detectable effect.

47. Answer: B

    Explanation: This task has potential exposure to hydrogen sulfide, methyl mercaptan, dimethyl sulfide, dimethyl disulfide, and sulfur dioxide. Bleaching operations produce chlorine and chlorine dioxide. *Source: Forest Products Chemistry. Papermaking Science and Technology*

48. Answer: B

    Explanation: A Chemical Hygiene Plan is a written program developed and implemented by the employer, which sets forth procedures, equipment, personal protective equipment, and work practices that are capable of protecting employees from the health hazards presented by hazardous chemicals used in the particular workplace. *Source: OSHA 29 CFR 1910.1450*

49. Answer: C

    Explanation: Absorbed lead is distributed initially to the blood and eventually to soft tissues (e.g., liver, kidneys, and other organs), and bone. *Source: Patty's Toxicology Volume 2, 5th Edition*

50. Answer A:

    Hazard: A condition, set of circumstances, or inherent property that can cause injury, illness, or death.
    Incident: An event in which a work-related injury or illness or fatality occurred or could have occurred
    Occupational Health and Safety Management System (OHSMS): A set of interrelated elements that establish and support occupational safety and health objectives.
    Risk: An estimate of the combination of the likelihood of an occurrence of a hazardous event or exposure, and the severity of the injury.

Self-Assessment Exam 4

1. A 10 mm cyclone with a pre-weighed filter is selected to sample for respirable particles. The flow rate was inadvertently set to 2.5 L/m. The flow rate for the type of cyclone used is 1.7 L/m. How will the incorrect flow rate effect the sample results?

   A) The capture of larger particles will increase.
   B) The only effect is overloading the filter more quickly.
   C) The capture of larger particles will decrease.
   D) The results must be corrected by multiplying by 0.32.

2. It is determined that 0.0027 mg of lead was collected on a filter. The pump operated from 0700 until 1420 without a break. The average flow rate was 1.93 L/m. What is the exposure expressed as an 8-hour time weighted average?

   A) $3.18 \ \mu g/m^3$
   B) $2.91 \ mg/m^3$
   C) $0.029 \ mg/m^3$
   D) $2.91 \ \mu g/m^3$

3. Select the most common media for active sampling for evaluating exposure to benzene:

   A) Activated charcoal tube.
   B) POVM.
   C) Treated silica gel tubes.
   D) Pre-weighed polyvinylchloride.

4. Spectrochemical monitors measure absorbance at the detector for a single compound. The absorbance is correlated to the chemical concentration through a concept known as:

   A) Bernoulli absorbance.
   B) Darcy-Wiesbach Law.
   C) Daltons Law.
   D) Beer Lambert Law.

5. Isokinetic sampling must be performed when sampling from a moving airstream, such as an exhaust stack or duct. Calculate the isokinetic flow rate for the following conditions: 37 mm cassette with a 2.5 mm opening sampling inside a 10-inch diameter duct with an airflow of $0.9 \ m^3/sec$. *Note*: the air flow is even across the duct.

   A) 3.3 L/min
   B) 5.2 L/min
   C) 6.5 L/min
   D) 7.6 L/min

6. When monitoring for BEIs, why is specimen collection time critical?

   A) Specimen collection is time sensitive and can yield an inconclusive result if collection takes too long.
   B) The airborne concentration of exposure could dissipate if specimen collection takes too long.
   C) All BEIs need to have a collection time of 5 minutes or less to be considered a valid sample.
   D) Rapid change of concentration in determinants is likely in some determinants.

7. The principle involved in neutron activation analysis consists of first irradiating a sample with neutrons in a nuclear reactor to produce specific radionuclides. Data reduction of _____ spectra then yields the concentrations of various elements in the samples being studied. With instrumental neutron activation analysis, it is possible to measure quantitatively about 60 elements in small samples.

   A) X-ray.
   B) Gamma ray.
   C) Microwave.
   D) Infrared.

8. What is the duration of the AIHA Lab Accreditation?

   A) 1 year.
   B) 2 years.
   C) 3 years.
   D) 4 years.

9. A method for analyzing contaminants with strong ions, including acids and bases is:

   A) Ion Chromatography.
   B) Gas Chromatography (GC).
   C) High Performance Liquid Chromatography (HPLC).
   D) Liquid Chromatography.

10. Which technique is not appropriate when collecting dust samples for x-ray diffraction analysis?

    A) PVC Filters.
    B) MCE Filters.
    C) Charcoal Tubes.
    D) Impingers.

11. Gas chromatography is used for analyzing volatile organic compounds or solvents. When a sample is in the GC column for analysis, what process accelerates the elution?

    A) GC Titration.
    B) GC Refraction.
    C) Heat in GC Oven.

D) Cool in GC Ice Bath.

12. Mass spectrometry (MS) is used in conjunction with _____ to identify the component that is responsible for a specific GC peak.

    A) High Performance Liquid Chromatography.
    B) Ion Chromatography.
    C) Liquid Chromatography.
    D) Gas Chromatography.

13. Choose the answer that correctly list the steps of a vision conservation program.

    A) Vision screening program, remedial program and professional fitting, and follow-up procedures.
    B) Vision screening program and fitting, and follow-up procedures.
    C) Environmental survey, vision screening program, remedial program, and professional fitting and follow-up procedures.
    D) Environmental survey, remedial program, and professional fitting and follow-up procedures.

14. Failure of the Eustachian tube to ventilate creates a vacuum in the middle ear space. This causes pathological events to occur. What is/are the pathological event(s)?

    A) Pulls fluid into the middle ear (Nonsuppurative otitis media).
    B) Pulls fluid out of the middle ear.
    C) Pulls the eardrum inward (retraction).
    D) Pulls the eardrum outward.
    E) A and B only.
    F) A and C only.
    G) All of the above.

15. Which of the following chemicals reacts dangerously with moisture in the air?

    A) Chlorine.
    B) Silane.
    C) Ammonia.
    D) Rhenium hexafluoride.

16. A crew is installing communications devices on top of a 13,000 feet tall mountain. Atmospheric pressure is 0.82 atm. Calculate the partial pressure for oxygen under these conditions.

    A) 632 Torr
    B) 209 Torr
    C) 130 Torr
    D) 90 Torr

17. The pressure in a closed vessel is doubled as a result of heating. The original temperature was 25°C. Calculate the new temperature.

    A) 50°C
    B) 596°K
    C) 461°R
    D) 250°K

18. What is the settling rate of vapor 3 inches below emission point for a solvent at STP, MW=-79 and SG of air-vapor mix = 1.0027?

    A) 20.3 ft/sec
    B) 0.2 ft/min
    C) 12.4 ft/min
    D) 0.00074 ft/sec

19. A prokaryote is a single-celled organism that lacks a membrane-bound nucleus (karyon), mitochondria, or any other membrane-bound organelle. Select the prokaryotic cell.

    A) Viruses.
    B) Protozoa.
    C) Bacteria.
    D) Ciliate.

20. Universal precautions apply to all of these fluids except:

    A) Amniotic fluid.
    B) Breast milk.
    C) Blood.
    D) Sweat containing blood.

21. Which of these methods should be used to determine the number of airborne colony forming units?

    A) Small-volume sampler.
    B) Large-volume sampler.
    C) Slit-to-agar impactor.
    D) Liquid impinger.

22. What are the four main categories of physical and chemical disinfection?

    A) Heat, liquid disinfectants, vapors and gasses, and radiation.
    B) Wet heat, dry heat, electrical current, and sunlight.
    C) Halogenated solvents, organic solvents, soaps, and carbamates.
    D) Alcohol, phenol, formaldehyde and glutaraldehyde.

23. Viruses are infectious agents that are not considered to be alive. Which of the following is not a characteristic of viruses?

A) Require a host.
B) Larger than bacteria.
C) Cannot replicate on their own.
D) Can generate particles called virions.

24. Choose the statement that best describes ionizing radiation decontamination.

A) Boil (212°F for > 30 minutes) and pasteurization (161°F for 15 seconds, or 143°F for 30 minutes) kills vegetative cells but not bacterial spores. High temperatures cause denaturation of enzymes and kill organisms.
B) Open flames and Bacti-Cinerators (tm) (an electrical device that dry-heats at 1600°F) are used to heat sterilize inoculation loops. Hot air ovens (160-180°C for 2 hours) are used for anhydrous materials (e.g., greases and powders). Incinerators are used to destroy infectious waste.
C) Inactivation of viruses, mycoplasma, bacteria, and fungi. Least effective and least perfected method of sterilization. Not practical as a disinfectant of liquids.
D) Sterilization of new, prepackaged medical devices (e.g., syringes and catheters) and in bulk package sterilization in the delivery of food industries.

25. The result of the percent mass of an air sample collected with an Anderson sampler (a cascade impactor) starting with stage 0 are 2.69, 5.56, 7.34, 22.00, 26.10, 23.67, 7.10, and 3.01 is presented in the table. What is the Geometric Standard Deviation (84.13% Method)?

A) 1.8 μm
B) 3.5 μm
C) 5.5 μm
D) 6.1 μm

Table: Geometric Standard Deviation (84.13% Method)

Stage Number	Size Range (μm)	Percent Mass	Cumulative % mass
Pre-collector		1.13	100
0	>9.0	2.69	98.87
1	5.8-9.0	5.56	96.18
2	4.7-5.8	7.34	90.62
3	3.3-4.7	22.00	83.28
4	2.1-3.3	26.10	61.28
5	1.1-2.1	23.67	35.18
6	0.7-1.1	7.10	11.51
7	0.4-0.7	3.01	4.41
Filter	0.0-0.4	1.40	1.40

The mass of particulate material collected on each stage is used to generate a cumulative mass distribution that can be plotted against a characteristic particle size for each stage. When the data is plotted on log-probability paper, the size below which 84.13% of the total particle mass falls is 4.8µm; and the size below which 50% of the particle mass falls is 2.6µm. Therefore, the GSD is the 84.13% value divided by the 50% value.

26. Calculate the cumulative error where the error measure is the coefficient of variation (CV). In the case where the CV_s is 5% (or 0.05) and the CV_a is 14% (or 0.14).

    A) 0.058
    B) 0.149
    C) 0.233
    D) 0.272

27. Choose the statement that correctly explains the confidence interval.

    A) I am 95% confident that the true mean is contained within the confidence interval.
    B) There is a 4.999% chance that the true mean is contained within the confidence interval.
    C) If an infinite number of samples were taken in the same manner, 95% of the time the true mean of the population would be contained within the confidence interval.
    D) If 1,000 samples were taken in the same manner, 100% of the time the true mean of the population would be contained within the confidence interval.

28. Choose the statement that best describes the arithmetic mean.

    A) A measure of central tendency, calculated as the sum of all values in a population divided by the number of values in the population.
    B) The exposure measurement that divides a set of measurements into two equal parts, with half less than and half greater than this value.
    C) The value in a set of measurements that occurs most frequently; the maximum value of a continuous probability density function.
    D) The positive square root of the variance of a distribution. It can be estimated from the slope of the straight line through data plotted on probability paper.

29. Choose the statement that best describes the lognormal distribution.

    A) An important symmetric probability distribution characterized completely by two parameters: the mean and the standard deviation. It has its highest ordinate at the center and tails off to zero in both directions, forming a bell-shaped curve.
    B) The sampling distribution of the mean approaches a normal distribution as the sample size increases, regardless of the shape of the underlying population distribution.
    C) The distribution of a random variable with the property such that the logarithms of its values are normally distributed.
    D) A quantity that describes a statistical population (e.g., mean and standard deviation, geometric mean, geometric standard deviation).

30. What is the prevalence rate of musculoskeletal injuries as of June 30, 2017 given:

- Population of workers at a construction on March 30, 2017 = 200,000
- Number of new active cases of musculoskeletal injuries occurring between January 1 and June 30, 2017 = 88
- Number of active musculoskeletal injuries on June 30, 2017 = 12

    A) 6 per 100,000 population.
    B) 12 per 100,000 population.
    C) 28 per 100,000 population.
    D) 73 per 100,000 population.

31. During stack sampling for particles, what is the effect on the results if the sample flow velocity is greater than the stack flow velocity?

    A) The measured concentration is greater than the actual concentration.
    B) The measured concentration is less than the actual concentration.
    C) The measured concentration is proportional to the square of the actual concentration.
    D) The measured concentration is equal to the actual concentration.

32. Concerning the Clean Air Act of 1970, what is the principal provision of section 171-192, Nonattainment areas?

    A) Gives detailed descriptions of what must be done in areas where NAAQS are not currently met.
    B) Lays out rules and regulations for regions with air cleaner than the NAAQS and for the protection of visibility, principally in the large national parks and wilderness areas.
    C) Establishes a federal acid deposition control program.
    D) Establishes the Standards of Performance for New Stationary Sources.

33. In terms of "isokinetic" sampling for particles:

    A) If the probe velocity is more than the stack velocity, then the measured concentration will be higher than the true stack concentration.
    B) If the probe velocity is more than the stack velocity, then the measured concentration will be lower than the true stack concentration.
    C) The probe velocity should be more than the stack velocity.
    D) The probe velocity should be less than the stack velocity.

34. What characterizes electrostatic precipitators?

    A) Increased efficiency as length of passage through precipitator increases.
    B) High efficiency, low cost, and high pressure drop.
    C) High efficiency for dry particles, not useful for wet particles.
    D) Increasing efficiency and pressure drop with time of operation.

35. You have been asked to assist a church pew manufacturer in the Ozark Mountains select a device for wood dust particle control. Select the most appropriate device.

    A) Venturi.
    B) Cyclone.
    C) Electrostatic precipitator.
    D) HEPA filter.

36. A researcher in a laboratory wants to add a fume hood to the laboratory. The hood has a 6-foot-wide sash, and it can be safely operated at sash height of 18 inches. The laboratory site safety manual stipulates that 80 FPM is the minimum allowable fume hood face velocity. Assuming a 10% safety factor, what is the minimum additional volume of make-up air to be supplied to the laboratory in order for the fume hood to function safely?

    A) 9 CFM
    B) 80 CFM
    C) 720 CFM
    D) 792 CFM

37. Mice have damaged a hose on a drum of a chemical in the storage room resulting in a leak and complete evaporation of the chemical. The technician notes that the airborne concentration in the room is 100 parts per million. The OEL is 5 parts per million. The room is 8 feet x 10 feet x 8 feet. The room is equipped with an exhaust fan that must be activated manually. Periodic maintenance records indicate the fan was exhausting 150 CFM one week ago. The IH wants to restrict entry until the level is 10% of the OEL. How long must workers wait until entering the room as allowed by the IH?

    A) 1.25 minutes.
    B) 22.6 minutes.
    C) 2.3 minutes.
    D) 12.5 minutes.

38. A 20 feet long section of 10-inch galvanized duct has a flow of 2000 CFM and a 20 feet long lection of 6-inch galvanized duct has a flow of 2000 CFM. Which of the ducts has the greatest SP loss?

    A) The 10-inch duct.
    B) The 6-inch duct.
    C) The loss is equal.
    D) There is no loss.

CIH Exam Study Workbook Volume II

39. Calculate the energy loss at a certain downstream point if the velocity pressure is 1.8 inches WG and the upstream static pressure is 2.0 inches WG.

   A) 0.001 inches WG
   B) 0.2 inches WG
   C) 0.6 inches WG
   D) 1.1 inches WG

40. A chemical hose manifold station is equipped with a collection trough. The trough is 16 inches from the front edge to the exhaust hood. The hood is 24 inches long and 6 inches wide and equipped with a flange. The average face velocity is 200 FPM. Calculate the capture velocity (centerline) at the front edge of the trough.

   A) 14.2 FPM
   B) 62 FPM
   C) 80.3 FPM
   D) 101 FPM

41. What is the standard static barometric pressure at sea level?

   A) 14.7 inches Hg
   B) 29.92 mm Hg
   C) 760 inches WG
   D) 407 inches WG

42. A manometer on the suction side of a fan is reading 0.58 inches WG velocity pressure and -1.2 inches WG static pressure. What is the total pressure on the suction side of the fan?

   A) -1.88 inches WG
   B) -0.62 inches WG
   C) 0.09 inches WG
   D) 1.24 inches WG

43. The term ergonomics can best be defined as:

   A) Designing equipment and tools for workers.
   B) Developing solutions to reduce work related injuries.
   C) The science of fitting workplace conditions to the capabilities of the working population.
   D) The anticipation, recognition, and control of workplace physical hazards.

44. The condition that results from insufficient blood supply, causing blanching and numbness in fingers is known as:

   A) Raynaud's Syndrome.
   B) Trigger finger.
   C) Boney Lacunae Syndrome.
   D) Femoral displacement.

190   *Copyright©2019 SPAN International Training, LLC*

45. When lifting a load, it is most important to:

   A) Lift from the side.
   B) Keep the load close to the body.
   C) Jerk the load to utilize internal forces.
   D) Take a deep breath.

46. Back belts:

   A) Are recommended by NIOSH.
   B) Are required by OSHA if back strain is possible.
   C) Have not been shown to lessen the risk of back injury among uninjured workers.
   D) Must be provided at no cost to employees who request them according to OSHA regulations.

47. When conducting sampling for the alcohol Cyclohexanol, what is the recommended media?

   A) Solid Sorbent tube.
   B) 1 μm PTFE filter.
   C) 5 μm Preweighed PVC filter.
   D) Silica Gel Tube.

48. What is the appropriate method when sampling for Silica, crystalline (as respirable dust)?

   A) NIOSH 5500.
   B) NIOSH 6890.
   C) NIOSH 6500.
   D) NIOSH 7500.

49. If it can be reasonable to conclude that the chemicals present in the workplace could add, one on the other, to the total effect, then it is also reasonable to consider adding the exposure assessment to derive a total exposure assessment. An example would be the presence of three chemicals, X, Y, and Z, with each having a similar toxicological effect on the same target organ. The total value (TV) is determined based on the concentration (C) and the threshold limit value (TLV) of each of the chemicals using the following equation:

$$TV = \frac{C_1}{TLV_1} + \frac{C_2}{TLV_2} + \cdots + \frac{C_n}{TLV_n}$$

Assume 30 ppm of acetone with a TLV of 250 ppm; 10 pm of toluene with a TLV of 20 ppm; and 110 ppm, of 2-propanol with a TLV of 200 ppm. Calculate the total value (TV).

   A) 0.40
   B) 0.74
   C) 1.17
   D) 1.46

50. The ACGIH recommends that TLVs not be used for which of the following?

    A) A legal limit.
    B) The exposure limit for healthy workers based on an 8-hour day, 40-hour week of work.
    C) As a guidance document.
    D) No recommendations are made by ACGIH.

51. Excursions in worker exposure levels may exceed ___ times the TLV-TWA for no more than a total of ___ minutes during a workday, and under no circumstances should they exceed ___ times the TLV-TWA, provided that the TLV-TWA is not exceeded.

    A) 5; 45; 3
    B) 3; 45; 5
    C) 3; 30; 10
    D) 3; 30; 5

52. An optical microscope is being used with the following conditions. Violet light (400 nm) is used to observe a sample under immersion oil. The sine of an angle for this microscope is 0.95. Calculate the theoretical limit of resolution.

    A) 0.18 μm
    B) 180 μm
    C) 257 nm
    D) 253 nm

53. Typically, the industrial or occupational hygienists have limited formal authority to accomplish their job tasks, although some may have positional authority. Accordingly, their role is described as management from a support position. Select the characteristics that describe the support role.

    A) Wide span of control
    B) More expertise than authority
    C) Viewed as a profit center
    D) Typically placed under Human Resources in the organizational structure

54. Select the best description of Participative Leadership.

    A) Direct people, explain decisions, and react to change.
    B) Build trust, facilitate decisions, and create a team identity.
    C) Involve people, develop individual performance, and resolve conflicts.
    D) Contain conflict, get input, and inspire teamwork.

55. Losses caused by radioactive materials are not covered by many insurance companies. In many experiments, a research laboratory creates radioisotopes for labeling purposes. If the manager for the company wants to minimize the potential loss associated with the radioisotopes, which method of controlling the risk avoids exposure to the loss?

A) Contract with another lab to perform all work requiring the use of radioisotopes.
B) Cap the maximum amount if radioisotopes allowed in the facility.
C) Transport the radioisotopes to a lab in another facility.
D) Implement, evaluate, and maintain a radiation health and safety program.

56. Assessment of performance, safety, health, durability, marketability, and social value should be conducted during what phase of Systems Development?

A) Identification.
B) Collection.
C) Analysis.
D) Implementation and evaluation.

57. Industrial Hygiene Audits:

A) Measure the effectiveness of industrial hygiene programs.
B) Should be conducted by persons with or without industrial hygiene expertise.
C) Contain an analysis of financial responsibilities and requirements of an industrial hygiene program.
D) Should be conducted before designing an industrial hygiene program.

58. ANSI Z-10, is an occupational safety management system. The system includes the Deming quality wheel. Select the answer that represents the elements of the continuous improvement process on the wheel.

A) Plan, Do, Confirm, Act.
B) Plan, Do, Check, Act.
C) Plan, Design, Confirm, Act.
D) Plan, Design, Create, Act.

59. You have been providing industrial hygiene support to a company since 1995. A change at the company results in a new safety officer, and the consulting contract goes to a different consulting firm. The senior IH from the new consulting firm requests your IH reports because the new safety officer cannot find any historical reports in his files. What is the best course of action?

A) Release the personal or business information to the new consultant.
B) Refuse to release the personal or business information.
C) Release the information after obtaining express authorization from the owner of the information.
D) Release the information only in hard copy format to prevent manipulation of the contents.

60. A sound level meter measures the noise of a machine at 100 dB at a distance of 5 feet. What is the noise level at a distance of 15 feet, assuming there are no other sources present and the measurements are conducted in a free field?

   A) 64 dB
   B) 71 dB
   C) 82 dB
   D) 90 dB

61. Company ABC plans to move five grinding stations into the same work area. Each grinding station measures 85 dB. Predict the approximate total SPL that will result.

   A) 80
   B) 82
   C) 90
   D) 92

62. If the lower frequency of an octave band is 55 Hz, what are the center and upper frequencies of this octave band?

   A) Center frequency = 71 Hz; Upper frequency= 100 Hz
   B) Center frequency = 78 Hz; Upper frequency= 110 Hz
   C) Center frequency = 84 Hz; Upper frequency= 129 Hz
   D) Center frequency = 90 Hz; Upper frequency= 148 Hz

63. A plant manager goes from a quiet office to the plant floor where loud noises are present. What type of occupational noise exposure does the plant manager encounter?

   A) Intermittent.
   B) Continuous.
   C) Impact.
   D) Peak.

64. Choose the answer that should not be recommended when conducting an audiometric test.

   A) Audiometric test should be pure tone.
   B) Audiometric test should be air conduction.
   C) Audiometric test should determine noise-induced hearing loss at the 8000-16000 Hz range.
   D) Audiometric test should test the minimum frequencies: 500, 1000, 2000, 3000, 4000, and 6000 Hz.

65. A maintenance shop has three pumps that operate continuously. The noise levels for the individual pumps are 90 dB, 95 dB and 101 dB. Select the most effective method for reducing noise levels in the shop.

   A) Eliminate the 90 and 95 dB machines.
   B) Eliminate the 95 dB machine.
   C) Eliminate the 101 dB machine.
   D) Eliminate the 90 dB machine.

66. OSHA requires protective footwear when hazards such as falling or rolling objects, penetration of the sole or electrical hazards exist. ANSI classifies footwear by impact and compression resistance. Conductive footwear would be worn as a control for what type of hazard?

    A) Electrocution.
    B) Thermal regulation.
    C) Static electricity discharge.
    D) Ergonomic injuries related to prolonged standing.

67. Which respirator has the highest assigned protection factor?

    A) Air-purifying respirator (APR)- half mask.
    B) Air-purifying respirator (APR)- full facepiece.
    C) Powered air-purifying respirator (PAPR)- half mask.
    D) Powered air-purifying respirator (PAPR)- full facepiece.

68. Fit testing should be performed for:

    A) Positive pressure respirators only.
    B) Negative pressure respirators only.
    C) All tight-fitting respirators.
    D) All respirators.

69. Which of the following would not be considered an acceptable administrative control for worker exposures to chemicals?

    A) Employee training.
    B) Worker rotation.
    C) Reduced work times.
    D) All are acceptable.

70. Calculate the wear time for a respirator user whose respirator use is required 6 hours of an 8- hour shift, but during this time, workers remove the mask for 2 minutes to wipe sweat from their face and the face shield.

    A) 100
    B) 98
    C) 97
    D) 96

71. Choose the answer that best describes an assigned protection factor (APF).

    A) The workplace level of respiratory protection that a respirator is expected to provide to employees when the employer implements a respirator protection program.
    B) A protection factor that defines the approximate duration it takes for a chemical to permeate through a specific pair of work gloves.
    C) A protection factor that defines the approximate duration it takes for a chemical to degrade through a specific pair of work gloves.
    D) The workplace level of respiratory protection that a respirator is expected to provide to employees approximately two months after the employer implements a respirator protection program. The safety professional must conduct baseline exposure monitoring before identifying an assigned protection factor for respirators.

72. Gamma rays originate in the nucleus and travel at the speed of light. This highly penetrating radiation interacts with matter in three ways. Select the answer that does not describe a method of interaction for gamma rays.

    A) Photoelectric effect.
    B) Pair production.
    C) Scintillation.
    D) Compton effect.

73. Select the term that refers to decay products of radioactive materials.

    A) Half-life.
    B) Activity.
    C) Progeny.
    D) Haploids.

74. A worker is exposed to a Radium source, which is an alpha emitter, with an estimated absorbed dose of 0.15 mrad/hour. Calculate the estimated dose equivalent for a 7-hour exposure.

Source	Quality Factor
X-ray	1.0
Gamma	1.0
Beta	1.0
Alpha	20
Slow neutron	10
Fast neutron	30

    A) 0.021 rem
    B) 0.02 mrem
    C) 3.0 mrem
    D) 0.003 rad

75. Radon is a noble gas that is linked to cancer in humans when exposed to high doses. Select the cancer related to Radon exposure.

    A) Brain.
    B) Leukemia.
    C) Ovarian.
    D) Lung.

76. The gamma radiation at 20 cm from an I-125 source is measured at 100 millirem/hour. The lead half-value layer is 0.0043 cm. What thickness of lead placed 20 cm from the source will lower the gamma radiation to 2 millirem/hour?

    A) 0.015 cm
    B) 0.024 cm
    C) 0.180 cm
    D) 0.400 cm

77. What is the function of an annular impactor head?

    A) Trap airborne particles.
    B) Collect airborne contamination.
    C) Collect surface contamination.
    D) Absorb liquid particles that are filterable.

78. How would you define a CW laser?

    A) A laser that emits radiation for a time less than 0.25 seconds.
    B) A laser that emits radiation for a time greater than or equal to 0.25 seconds.
    C) A laser that promotes a human aversion response to UV radiation.
    D) A laser that promotes a human aversion response to IR radiation.

79. Which of the following is/are the main damage mechanism(s) from lasers?

    A) Photomechanical.
    B) Photomechanical and Thermal.
    C) Photomechanical and Photochemical.
    D) Photomechanical, Thermal and Photochemical.

80. Which of the following are chronic skin effects associated with UV exposure?

    A) Photokeratitis.
    B) Aging of the skin, skin cancer, and photosensitization.
    C) Hair movement, shock and burns.
    D) Erythema and photostimulation.

81. "Arc eye" or "welder's flash" is a result from high-intensity exposure to UV-B and UV-C. This injury results from exposure of the unprotected eye to a welding arc or other artificial sources rich in UV-B and UV-C. What is the medical condition for "arc eye" or "welder's flash?"

    A) Photokeratitis and Photoconjunctivitis.
    B) Traumatic Iritis.
    C) Corneal abrasion.
    D) Subconjunctival Hemorrhage.

82. Key characteristics of light sources are efficiency, color rendering index, and color temperature. Choose the answer below that correctly defines efficiency in relation to light sources.

    A) A relative scale that rates how perceived colors of objects illuminated by a given source matches the color produced by the same object when illuminated by a reference standard light source.
    B) The ability of converting energy to visible light.
    C) The ability of converting visible light to energy.
    D) The color of a blackbody radiator at a given temperature.

83. Welding curtains may be made of materials that are either opaque or transparent to visible wavelengths. Choose the answer that correctly states why transparent welding curtains are utilized in an industrial setting?

    A) Allows easier communication with employees and management can keep an eye on employees.
    B) Increases productivity and allows visual contact with welders.
    C) Lowers the airborne concentration of welding fumes and provides an increase of general illumination levels.
    D) Allows visual contact with welders, reduces arc glare, and increases general illumination levels.

84. Which of the following best describes conduction?

    A) The transfer of heat between two objects using electromagnetic radiation.
    B) The transfer of heat by air movement or air currents.
    C) The transfer of heat from cooler to warmer objects.
    D) The transfer of heat when two objects come into contact.

85. What condition is characterized by red papules in areas where clothing contacts skin and may be caused as excess sweat is absorbed by the keratinous layer of the skin?

    A) Heat cramps.
    B) Measles.
    C) Prickly heat.
    D) Rocky Mountain Spotted Fever.

86. What are some signs and symptoms of heat exhaustion?

    A) Fatigue, nausea, headache, giddiness. Skin clammy and pale.
    B) Painful spasms of muscles used during work. Onset during or after work hours.
    C) Hot, dry skin. Rectal temperature above 40.5°C. Confusion, loss of consciousness, convulsions.
    D) Miliaria rubra and Miliaria profunda.

87. Rank the following heat stress conditions in order from most severe to least severe.

    A) Heat rash, heat stroke, heat cramps.
    B) Heat cramps, heat rash, heat stroke.
    C) Heat cramps, heat exhaustion, heat stroke.
    D) Heat stroke, heat exhaustion, heat cramps.

88. Assuming the following conditions, what is the WBGT index for a day shift employee who is working outside for the entire shift:

    - Wet Bulb Temperature = 26°C
    - Globe Temperature = 35°C
    - Dry Bulb Temperature = 30°C

    A) 28°C
    B) 30°C
    C) 34°C
    D) 38°C

89. The skin notation in the ACGIH-TLV booklet indicates:

    A) The potential for skin damage exists.
    B) Will cause skin sensitization.
    C) Potential skin carcinogen.
    D) Exposure may occur via the cutaneous route.

90. What is the largest organ of the body?

    A) Skin.
    B) Lung.
    C) Heart.
    D) Brain.

91. Which of the following is not associated with decreased sperm count in humans?

    A) Ethylene dibromide.
    B) Dibromochloropropane.
    C) Formaldehyde.
    D) Lead.

92. The dose of a chemical agent reaching a target organ is best described as a function of:

   A) The location of the organ and the size of the organ.
   B) The duration of exposure and concentration of exposure.
   C) The size of the organ and concentration of exposure.
   D) The mass and molecular weight of the chemical.

93. Which of the following is best described by the statement "any cutaneous abnormality resulting from, or aggravated by, factors in the occupational environment?"

   A) Sensitizers.
   B) Occupational dermatitis.
   C) Occupational dermatoses.
   D) Contact dermatitis.

94. Which of the following is not associated with "hard metal disease," with symptoms of metaplasia of bronchial epithelium as well as pulmonary fibrosis?

   A) Aluminum.
   B) Titanium.
   C) Tungsten.
   D) Tantalum.

95. Metal working fluids are used to reduce heat and friction, thereby improving product quality in the machining process. There are several formulations of metal working fluids, one of which is called straight oil. Straight oil is best described as:

   A) Synthetic fluid.
   B) Petroleum fluid.
   C) Water based fluid.
   D) Semi-synthetic fluid.

96. A manufacturing facility in a rural area uses chlorinated solvents in tanks to degrease parts. There is also plasma cutting and shaping of steel, as well as extruding plastic parts. Some of the employees have cattle farms. These workers were discussing that they smelled something like freshly cut hay in the building. They felt it was odd since no one was cutting hay at this time of year. What may be the source of this odor?

   A) The photo-oxidation and thermal decomposition of chlorinated hydrocarbons.
   B) The biological decomposition of stored hay.
   C) The production of ozone.
   D) The thermal decomposition of plasticizers.

97. Caisson workers are often exposed to extreme conditions, such as reduced natural ventilation, low light, and the potential for fires and explosions. Workers must also watch for loose soil and rock. Being struck by moving loading or hauling equipment and flying debris is possible. In addition, there are limited means of access and egress and potential exposure to dangerous gases, such as hydrogen sulfide. Work may be conducted in confined spaces, in compressed air, or near electrical, drilling and blasting sites. Select an occupational illness associated with caisson work.

A) Decompression sickness.
B) Pneumoconiosis.
C) Phossy jaw.
D) Reichel's syndrome.

98. Worker protection is recommended when dealing with mold remediation. What is the minimum level of protection in work areas with up to 100ft2 of mold?

A) No work protection is necessary.
B) Disposable respirator (e.g., N-95) and gloves.
C) Fit-tested respirators with High Efficiency Particulate Air (HEPA) cartridges, coveralls, and gloves.
D) Self-Contained Breathing Apparatus (SCBA).

99. Choose the statement that best describes a confined space.

A) Is large enough and so configured that an employee cannot enter it to perform assigned work.
B) Has limited or restricted means for entry.
C) Has limited or restricted means for exit only.
D) Is designed for continuous employee occupancy.

100. What are the primary sources of occupational lead exposure?

A) Workplace air and surface dust.
B) Workplace air and ground sources.
C) Surface dust and ground sources.

Self-Assessment Exam 4 Answers

1. Answer: C
   Explanation:
   The centrifugal force exerted on the larger particles exerted by the increase in airflow will force them out of the airstream and allow only smaller particles onto the filter. This sample is considered invalid.

2. Answer: D
   Explanation:
   Calculate sample time: $T = 440$ minutes

   Calculate sample volume:
   $$FR \times T = V$$

$$1.93 \text{ L/m x } 440 \text{ minutes} = 849.2 \text{ L}$$

Calculate sample concentration:

$$\frac{0.0027 \text{ mg}}{849.2 \text{ L}} \left(\frac{1000 \text{ L}}{m^3}\right)\left(\frac{1000 \text{ ug}}{mg}\right) = 3.18 ug/m^3$$

Calculate the 8-hour TWA:

$$\frac{3.18 \times 440}{480} = 2.91 \ ug/m^3$$

3. Answer: A
   Explanation: NIOSH 1501 GC/FD is the method recommended for benzene.

4. Answer: D
   Explanation: Beer-Lambert Law (also known as Beer's Law) states that there is a linear relationship between the absorbance and the concentration of a sample. For this reason, Beer's Law can *only* be applied when there is a linear relationship. Beer's Law is written as:

$$A=\epsilon lc$$

   Source: Fundamentals of Industrial Hygiene 6th ed. NSC. UC Davis on-line chemistry lecture

5. Answer: B
   Explanation:

   For isokinetic sampling: $\frac{Q_{sample}}{Q_{duct}} = \left[\frac{D_{sample}}{D_{duct}}\right]^2$

   Where:
   Q_{sample} is the air flow at the sample probe (m³/sec).
   Q_{duct} is the air flow inside the duct (m³/sec).
   D_{sample} is the probe opening diameter (cm).
   D_{duct} is the duct diameter (cm).

   Step 1: Convert the duct diameter to cm and sample opening diameter to cm
   10 inches x 2.54 cm/inch = 25.4 cm
   2.5 mm x 1 cm/10 mm = 0.25 cm

   Step 2: Convert the duct flow to L/min
   0.9 m³/sec x 1000 L/m³ x 60 sec/min = 54000 L/min

   Step 3: Solve for Q_{sample}

$$\frac{Q_{sample}}{Q_{duct}} = \left[\frac{D_{sample}}{D_{duct}}\right]^2$$

$$\frac{Q_{sample}}{54000 L/min_{duct}} = \left[\frac{0.25\ cm_{sample}}{25.4\ cm_{duct}}\right]^2$$

$$Q_{sample} = 0.000096875 \times 54000 \text{ L/min}$$

$$Q_{sample} = 5.2 \text{ L/min}$$

6. Answer: D

   Explanation: Because the concentration of some determinants can change rapidly, the specimen collection time (sampling time) is very important and must be observed and recorded carefully. The sampling time is specified in the BEI and is determined by the duration of retention of the determinant. Substances and determinants that accumulate may not require a specific sampling time. *Source: TLVs and BEIs Based on Documentation of the Threshold Limit Values for Chemical Substances and Physical Agents and Biological Exposure Indices.*

7. Answer: B

   Explanation: After the irradiation, the characteristic gamma rays emitted by the decaying radionuclides are quantitatively measured by gamma spectroscopy, where the gamma rays detected at a particular energy are indicative of a specific radionuclide's presence. Also, x-rays do not originate in the nucleus. *Source: Cornell University, Ward Center for Nuclear Sciences*

8. Answer: B

   Explanation: The accreditation duration is 2 years per the AIHA Lab Accreditation Program LLC – module 3. This program has been in operation for more than 30 years.

9. Answer: A

   Explanation: Ion chromatography is used for simultaneous and sequential analysis of ions including fluorine ion, chlorine ion, bromine ion, sulfate ion, sulfite ion, nitrate ion, nitrite ion, and phosphate ion. *Source: The Occupational Environment: Its Evaluation, Control and Management, 3rd edition*

10. Answer: C

    Explanation: Charcoal tubes is not a technique to collect dust samples for x-ray diffraction. Impingers, MCE Filters and PVC Filters are techniques that can be used to collect dust samples for x-ray diffraction analysis. It may be required to re-suspend the dust or ash the filters, and deposit it on an appropriate silver membrane surface for analysis.

11. Answer: C

    Explanation: Gas chromatography is the proper technique for analyzing volatile organic compounds or solvents. A sample is injected into a hot injector port of a gas chromatograph, where it is volatilized and carried through a very long and narrow GC column with the aid of a carrier gas (e.g., helium). The mixture of compounds is separated by the GC column. During the separation, the GC column is heated in a GC oven under controlled conditions to volatilize the compounds and accelerate the elution. The compounds eluting from the GC column are then passed through a detector. The detector response is monitored, resulting in a chromatogram. *Source: Applications and Computational Elements of Industrial Hygiene*

12. Answer: D

    Explanation: Mass spectrometry (MS) is used in conjunction with gas chromatography (GC) to identify the component that is responsible for a specific GC peak. The GC separates the mixture into components. The individual components then are analyzed by MS. MS fractures and ionizes the compounds, and then accelerates and separates them based on charge/mass ratio. *Source: Applications and Computational Elements of Industrial Hygiene*

13. Answer: C

    Explanation: Vision Conservation Program consists of four steps. These steps include environmental survey, vision screening program, remedial program, and professional fitting and follow-up procedures. *Source: Fundamentals of Industrial Hygiene 5th Edition*

14. Answer: F

    Explanation: Failure of the Eustachian tube to ventilate creates a vacuum in the middle ear space, which in turn causes one of two pathological events to occur: It pulls fluid into the middle ear, resulting in a condition called nonsuppurative otitis media, or it pulls the eardrum inward (retraction). *Source: Fundamentals of Industrial Hygiene 5th edition*

15. Answer: D. **Explanation:** Rhenium hexafluoride reacts with water to produce hydrofluoric acid. *Source: Fundamentals of Industrial Hygiene 5th edition*

16. Answer: C
    Explanation:

    Step 1: Convert the current pressure to Torr

    $$0.82 \text{ atm} \times \frac{760 \, Torr}{1 \, atm} = 623.2 \text{ Torr}$$

    Step 2: Calculate the partial pressure in Torr

    Oxygen is 20.9% of the atmosphere
    0.209 x 623.2 Torr = 130 Torr

17. Answer: B
    Explanation: The volume remains constant.
    Step 1: Convert temperature to absolute

    $$25 + 273 = 298°K$$

    Step 2: Solve for T

    $$\frac{P_1}{T_1} = \frac{P_2}{T_2}$$

$$\frac{1}{298} = \frac{2}{X}$$

$$X = 298 \times 2$$

$$X = 596$$

18. Answer: C

    Explanation: Assume mixing and stack height are inconsequential. If distance of falling height is less than 1 foot, then:

$$V_s = \sqrt{\frac{2g \, (SG - 1)(n)}{SG}}$$

Where

    V_s is setting rate (ft/sec).
    g is gravitational acceleration (ft/sec^2).
    h is distance from source (feet).
    SG is the specific gravity of the mixture.

$$V_s = \sqrt{\frac{2\left(32 \frac{ft}{sec^2}\right)(.0027)(.25ft)}{1.0027}}$$

$$= \sqrt{.0430836}$$

$$= .208 \text{ ft/sec}$$

Convert to feet/min

.208 ft/sec x 60sec/min = 12.4 ft/min

19. Answer: C

Explanation: Prokaryotes are cellular organisms that do not have a nuclear membrane. Found in the kingdom Monera as bacteria and blue-green algae. *Cell Biology, 2nd ed., Pollard et al.*

20. Answer: B

Explanation: Universal precautions apply to blood, fluids in which blood is indistinguishably mixed, and bodily fluids that visibly contain blood; however, breast milk is excluded from universal precautions unless it visibly contains blood.

21. Answer: C

Explanation: The slit to agar method is the best choice.

22. Answer: A

Explanation: Heat, liquid disinfectants, vapors and gasses, and radiation are the four main categories. Wet and dry heat are forms of heat utilized. Halogens, organic solvents and soaps are types of disinfectants. Carbamates are a type of pesticide. *Source: AIHA Biohazards Reference Manual*

23. Answer: B

Explanation: Viruses are smaller than bacteria (<30nm). Virions are particles of genetic material, proteins and lipids. *Source: Intermountain Healthcare Biohazard Lecture*

24. Answer: D

Table: Physical Agent Decontamination Techniques and Process/Application

Technique	Process/Application
Steam	Heat at 250°F under pressure (15-18 psi) in an autoclave. Most widely used and convenient method of sterilization.
Wet Heat	Boil (212°F for > 30 minutes) and pasteurization (161°F for 15 seconds, or 143°F for 30 minutes) kills vegetative cells but not bacterial spores. High temperatures cause denaturation of enzymes and kill organisms.
Dry Heat	Open flames and Bacti-Cinerators (tm) (an electrical device that dry-heats at 1600°F) are used to heat sterilize inoculation loops. Hot air ovens (160-180°C for 2 hours) are used for anhydrous materials (e.g., greases and powders). Incinerators are used to destroy infectious waste.
Ionizing Radiation	Sterilization of new, prepackaged medical devices (e.g., syringes and catheters) and in bulk package sterilization in the delivery of food industries.
Ultraviolet (UV) Radiation	Inactivation of viruses, mycoplasma, bacteria, and fungi. Least effective and least perfected method of sterilization. Not practical as a disinfectant of liquids.
Filtration	Membrane filters are used to remove bacteria, yeast, and molds from biologic and pharmaceutical solutions. Common spore sizes: 0.22µm, 0.45µm, and 0.8µm

25. Answer: A

Explanation:

Table: Geometric Standard Deviation (84.13% Method)

Stage Number	Size Range (μm)	Percent Mass	Cumulative % mass
Pre-collector		1.13	100
0	>9.0	2.69	98.87
1	5.8-9.0	5.56	96.18
2	4.7-5.8	7.34	90.62
3	3.3-4.7	22.00	83.28
4	2.1-3.3	26.10	61.28
5	1.1-2.1	23.67	35.18
6	0.7-1.1	7.10	11.51
7	0.4-0.7	3.01	4.41
Filter	0.0-0.4	1.40	1.40

The mass of particulate material collected on each stage is used to generate a cumulative mass distribution that can be plotted against a characteristic particle size for each stage. When the data is plotted on log-probability paper, the size below which 84.13% of the total particle mass falls is 4.8μm, and the size below which 50% of the particle mass falls is 2.6μm. Therefore, the GSD is the 84.13% value divided by the 50% value.

Table: Geometric Standard Deviation (84.13% Method)

Stage Number	Size Range (μm)	Percent Mass	Cumulative % mass
Pre-collector		1.13	100
0	>9.0	2.69	98.87
1	5.8-9.0	5.56	96.18
2	4.7-5.8	7.34	90.62
3	3.3-4.7	22.00	83.28
4	2.1-3.3	26.10	61.28
5	1.1-2.1	23.67	35.18
6	0.7-1.1	7.10	11.51
7	0.4-0.7	3.01	4.41
Filter	0.0-0.4	1.40	1.40

Calculate the Geometric Standard Deviation (84.13% Method)

$$GSD = \frac{84.13\ \%tile\ value}{50\ \%tile\ value}$$

$$GSD = \frac{84.13\%}{50\%}$$

$$GSD = \frac{4.8\mu m}{2.6\mu m}$$

$$GSD = 1.8\ \mu m$$

Source: Industrial-Occupational Hygiene Calculations: A Professional Reference

26. Answer: B

Explanation: Calculate the cumulative error.

$$CV_T = \sqrt{(CV_s)^2 + (CV_a)^2}$$

$$CV_T = \sqrt{[(0.05)^2 + (0.14)^2]}$$

$$CV_T = 0.149$$

Source: Industrial-Occupational Hygiene Calculations: A Professional Reference

27. Answer: C

Explanation: The interpretation of the confidence interval is as follows: if an infinite number of samples were taken in the same manner, 95% of the time the true mean μ of the population would be contained within the confidence interval. It does not mean that you have 95% confidence that the true mean μ is contained in that particular confidence interval. *Source: Industrial-Occupational Hygiene Calculations: A Professional Reference*

28. Answer: A

Explanation: Arithmetic mean - A measure of central tendency, calculated as the sum of all values in a population divided by the number of values in the population. *Source: Industrial-Occupational Hygiene Calculations: A Professional Reference*

29. Answer: C

Explanation: Lognormal distribution - The distribution of a random variable with the property such that the logarithms of its values are normally distributed. *Source: Industrial-Occupational Hygiene Calculations: A Professional Reference*

30. Answer A

Explanation: Calculate the prevalence.

$$\text{Prevalence} = \frac{\text{total number of cases of a disease at a given time}}{\text{total popuation at risk at a given time}}$$

$$\text{Prevalence} = \frac{12}{200,000} = 0.00006 \times 100,000 = 6.0 \text{ per } 100,000 \text{ population}$$

Source: Epidemiology 5th Edition, Leon Gordis

31. Answer: A

Explanation: Isokinetic sampling is required to obtain measured results equal to the actual concentration.

32. Answer: A
Explanation:

Sections of the Clean Air Act of 1970, as Amended in 1977 and 1990

Section	Title	Principal Provisions
107	Air Quality Control Regions (AQCR)	Divides the country into regions. States must administer air quality in each such region, under federal supervision.
109	National Ambient Air Quality Standards (NAAQS)	Establishes National Ambient Air Quality Standards.
110	State Implementation Plans (SIP)	Requires states to prepare and enforce State Implementation Plans. Gives details on how it has to be done.
111	New Source Performance Standards (NSPS)	Establishes the Standards of Performance for New Stationary Sources.
112 and 301-306	National Emission Standards for Hazardous Air Pollutants (NESHAP)	Establishes National Emission Standards for Hazardous Air Pollutants, also called air toxics.
160-169	Prevention of Significant Deterioration (PSD)	Lays out rules and regulations for regions with air cleaner than the NAAQS and for the protection of visibility, principally in the large national parks and wilderness areas.
171-192	Nonattainment areas	Gives detailed descriptions of what must be done in areas where NAAQS are not currently met.
202-235	Mobile sources	Places control on motor vehicle emissions mostly in the hands of the federal government; sets motor vehicle and fuel composition standards.
401-416	Acid deposition control	Establishes a federal acid deposition control program.
601-618	Stratospheric ozone protection	Establishes programs for protection of the stratospheric ozone layer.

Source: US EPA

33. Answer: B
Explanation: Isokinetic sampling is required for particles in stacks. If the sampling velocity is greater than the velocity in the stack, the measured concentration is greater than the actual concentration. If the sample velocity is less than the velocity in the stack, the measured concentration is less than the actual concentration. If the sample velocity is equal to the velocity in the stack, the measured concentration is equal to the actual concentration.
Source: Industrial Hygiene Reference and Study Guide, 3rd edition

34. Answer: A
Explanation: As particles are collected on the proximal collectors they become less effective; however, if more collectors follow, then more particles will be collected. A longer path allows for more collectors. *Source: Air Pollution Control Engineering, 2nd Edition*

35. Answer: B
Explanation: The cyclone is frequently used in wood shops to remove dust particles from the air. The venture is a high maintenance device that is effective for small particles. Precipitators are energy intense and better suited for fine particles. HEPA filters are best suited for small particles and would be subject to frequent overloading and maintenance issues. *Industrial Hygiene Reference and Study Guide. 3rd Edition*

36. Answer: D
Explanation: Known

$$V = 80 \text{ FPM}$$
$$A = (6\text{ft. X } 1.5\text{ft}) = 9 \text{ ft}^2$$

$$Q = VA$$

$$Q = 1.1 \, x \, (80 \, fpm \, x \, 9 \, ft^2)$$

$$Q = 792 \, CFM$$

37. Answer: B
Explanation:
Step 1: Calculate the target concentration, C_2

$$0.10 \text{ x } 5 \text{ PPM} = 0.5 \text{ PPM}$$

Step 2: Calculate the room volume

$$V_r = 8 \text{ x } 10 \text{ x } 8 = 640 \text{ ft}^3$$

Step 3: Solve for $t_2 - t_1$, which is known as Δt

$$t_2 - t_1 = -\frac{V_r}{Q'} ln\left(\frac{C_2}{C_1}\right)$$

$$\Delta t = -\frac{640 \, ft^3}{150 \, cfm} ln\left(\frac{0.5 \, ppm}{100 \, ppm}\right)$$

$$\Delta t = -4.266 \text{ x } -5.298$$

$$= 22.6 \text{ minutes}$$
Source: Industrial Occupational Hygiene Calculations: A Professional Reference

38. Answer: B

     Explanation: Conceptually, if the same volume is passing through a smaller duct, the gas is moving faster and having more losses due to friction, turbulence, etc.

     Mathematically, the SP_{loss} for the 10-inch duct is 0.41 inches WG. The SP_{loss} for the 6-inch duct is 3.1 inches WG.

$$SP_{loss} = \frac{K}{100\ ft}\ x\ VP\ x\ length\ ft$$

39. Answer: B

     Explanation:

$$SP_1 + VP_1 = SP_2 + VP_2 + h_L$$

$$SP_2 = 2.0\ inches\ WG$$
$$VP_2 = 1.8\ inches\ WG$$

     Step 1: Rearrange the equation

$$Since,\ SP_1 = SP_2\ and\ VP_1\ and\ VP_1 = VP_2,\ then$$

$$SP_2 = -VP_2 - h_L$$

     Step 2: Solve for h_L

$$h_L = -SP_2 - VP_2$$

$$h_L = -(-2.0\ inches\ WG) - 1.8\ inches\ WG$$

$$h_L = 0.2\ inches\ WG$$

40. Answer: A

     Explanation:
     Step 1: Determine the hood type and formula to use for capture velocity

$$The\ aspect\ ratio\ is\ \frac{width}{length} = \frac{6\ inches}{24\ inches} = 0.25$$

     By definition, if the aspect ratio is greater than 0.2, then the hood is a flanged hood, then according to ACGIH:

$$Q = 0.75V(10X^2 + A)$$

     Note: L & X are expressed as feet and V as feet/minute

     Step 2: Solve for Q at the hood opening

$$Q = VA$$

     Note: A = L x W expressed as feet = 1 ft^2

$$Q = 200 \, FPM \, x \left(\frac{6 \, inches}{12 \, \frac{inches}{foot}} \, x \, \frac{24 \, inches}{12 \, \frac{inches}{foot}} \right)$$

$$Q = 200 \, \text{CFM}$$

Step 3: Solve for V

$$Q = 0.75V \, x \, (10X^2 + A)$$

$$200 \, \text{CFM} = 0.75V \, x \, \left(10\left(\frac{16 \, inches}{12\frac{inches}{foot}}\right)^2 + 1 \, ft^2\right)$$

$$\frac{200 \, CFM}{0.75 \, x \, 18.78 \, ft^2} = V$$

$$14.2 \, \text{FPM} = V$$

ACGIH Industrial Ventilation: A Manual of Recommended Practice, 24th Edition

41. Answer: D
    Explanation:
    Standard static pressure: 29.92 inches Hg = 760 mm Hg = 407 inches WG. Therefore, if a fan creates a -1 inches WG, then the absolute pressure is 406 inches WG. *Source: IH Workbook, 6th edition, Burton*

42. Answer: B
    Explanation:

$$TP = VP + SP$$

VP = 0.58 inches WG
SP = -1.2 inches WG

Step 1: Solve for TP

$$TP = VP + SP$$

$$TP = 0.58 \, inches \, WG \, + (-1.2 \, inches \, WG)$$

$$TP = \, -0.62 \, inches \, WG$$

Source: Industrial-Occupational Hygiene Calculations: A Professional Reference

43. Answer: C

    Explanation: The science of fitting the task or conditions to the worker has been the historical definition. The AIHA Ergonomics committee defines ergonomics as 'A multidisciplinary science that applies to principles based on the physical and psychological capabilities of people to the design or modification of jobs, equipment, products and work places.' *Source: The Occupational Environment, Its Evaluation, Control, and Management. 3rd edition*

44. Answer: A

    Explanation: Trigger finger is a type of tenosynovitis in which the tendon becomes locked or nearly locked, so that forced movement is jerky. Raynaud's is also known as vibration syndrome and white finger syndrome. *Source: The Occupational Environment, Its Evaluation, Control, and Management. 3rd edition*

45. Answer: B

    Explanation: When lifting a load, it is important to do all of the following: securely grip the load, keep the load close to the body, use a comfortable posture, lift slowly and evenly, and do not twist the back. *Source: NIOSH/CDC*

46. Answer: C

    Explanation: The use of lifting belts for professional material handling does not seem to be an effective way of preventing overexertion injuries. When preparing to lift or lower a load, we instinctively develop intra-abdominal pressure within the trunk cavity. The pressure is believed to help support the curvature of the spine during the lifting or lowering effort. An external wrapping around the abdominal region might help to maintain the internal pressure because it makes the walls of the pressure column stiffer. A large number of studies have been performed, summarized, and reviewed by McGill (1999), Lavender, et al (1998), and Thoumier, et al (1998). Their conclusions neither summarily support nor condemn the wearing of support belts in industrial jobs. *Source: Fundamentals of Industrial Hygiene 5th Edition*

47. Answer: A

    Explanation: According to the NIOSH Manual of Analytical Methods, method 1402, the recommended media when sampling for Cyclohexanol is a solid sorbent tube (coconut shell). The analysis is done via gas chromatography-FID. *Source: NIOSH Manual of Analytical Methods 4th edition*

48. Answer: D

    Explanation: According to the NIOSH Manual of Analytical Methods, the appropriate method when sampling for Silica, crystalline (as respirable dust) is NIOSH 7500. This requires the use of a cyclone and pre-weighed PVC filter. The analysis is done by x-ray diffraction. *Source: NIOSH Manual of Analytical Methods 4th edition*

49. Answer: C
Explanation:
Step 1: Solve for TV

$$TV = \frac{C_1}{TLV_1} + \frac{C_2}{TLV_2} + \cdots + \frac{C_n}{TLV_n}$$

$$TV = \frac{30}{250} + \frac{10}{20} + \frac{110}{200}$$

$$TV = 0.12 + 0.5 + 0.55$$

$$TV = 1.17$$

The general standard for total value is 1.00. It could be judged from this evaluation that the exposure may have an additive impact above acceptable limits, and the exposure should be reduced. *Source: The Occupational Environment: Its Evaluation, Control and Management 3rd edition, Vol. 1*

50. Answer: A
Explanation: The ACGIH TLV is a recommended limit for use by professionals in the health and safety profession. *Source: ACGIH TLV and BEI publication*

51. Answer: D
Explanation: Excursions in worker exposure levels may exceed 3 times the TLV-TWA for no more than a total of 30 minutes during a workday, and under no circumstances should they exceed 5 times the TLV-TWA, provided that the TLV-TWA is not exceeded. *Source: TLVs and BEIS Based on the Documentation of the Threshold Limit Values for Chemical Substances and Physical Agents & Biological Exposure Indices*

52. Answer: A
Explanation:

Step 1: Solve for d

$$d = \frac{0.61\lambda}{\eta sin\alpha}$$

$$d = \frac{0.61 \ x \ 400nm}{1.52 \ x \ 0.95}$$

$$d = 178 \text{ nm or } 0.18 \text{ μm}$$

53. Answer: B

Explanation: In addition to more expertise than authority, G. Bellman identifies the following characteristics in the book, "Getting Things Done When You Are Not In Charge:" important influence but not final authority, free access to the organization, regular interaction with people of greater authority, planning is difficult, may not understand the big picture, viewed as a cost center. *Source: The Occupational Environment: It's Evaluation, Control, and Management, 3rd Edition*

54. Answer: C

Explanation:

Supervisory leadership: Direct people, explain decisions, react to change, contain conflict.

Team leadership: Build trust, facilitate decisions, create a team identity, foresee and influence change, build trust, and inspire teamwork.

Participative leadership: Involve people, develop individual performance, resolve conflicts, get input, and develop individual performance. *Source: The Occupational Environment: It's Evaluation, Control, and Management, 3rd Edition*

55. Answer: A

Explanation: Contracting with another lab to perform work requiring the use of radioisotopes is termed risk transfer. It is the only solution to completely avoid exposure.

56. Answer: D

Explanation: Performance, safety, health, durability, marketability, and social value should be assessed at the implementation and evaluation phase of Systems Development.

57. Answer: A

Explanation: An industrial hygiene audit measures the effectiveness of an industrial hygiene program.

58. Answer: B

Explanation: The American National Standards Institute, in conjunction with ASSE produced, Z10. Elements include Management Leadership, Employee Participation, Planning, System Implementation, Evaluation-Corrective Actions, and Management Review. *Source: Industrial Hygiene Reference and Study Guide, 3rd Edition*

59. Answer: C

Explanation: The Cannon of 1995 contains the interpretive guideline that states, "Industrial Hygienists should release confidential personal or business information only with the information owners' express authorization, except when there is a duty to disclose information as required by law or regulation." *Source: 1995 Cannon of Industrial Hygiene Ethical Conduct*

60. Answer: D
   Explanation:

$$SPL_2 = SPL_1 + 20 \, log\left(\frac{d_1}{d_2}\right)$$

$$SPL_1 = 100 \, dB$$
$$d_1 = 5 \, feet$$
$$d_2 = 15 \, feet$$

Step 1: Solve for SPL$_2$

$$SPL_2 = 100 \, dB + 20 \, log\left(\frac{5 \, feet}{15 \, feet}\right)$$

$$SPL_2 = 100 \, dB + 20 \, log(0.33)$$

$$SPL_2 = 100 \, dB - 9.6$$

$$SPL_2 = 90 \, dB$$

Source: Industrial-Occupational Hygiene Calculations: A Professional Reference

61. Answer: D
   Explanation:

$$SPL_f = SPL_l + 10 \, log(n)$$

Step 1: Solve for SPL$_f$

$$SPL_f = 85 + log(5)$$

$$SPL_f = 85 + 10 \, (0.699)$$

$$SPL_f = 92.0$$

Source: Occupational Safety Calculations: A Professional Reference, 2nd Edition

62. Answer: B
Explanation:

$$f_2 = \sqrt{2f_1}$$

Step 1: Calculate the center frequency of the octave band

$$Center\ frequency = \sqrt{2}(55)$$

$$Center\ frequency = 78\ Hz$$

Step 1: Calculate the center frequency of the octave band

$$Upper\ frequency = \sqrt{2}(78)$$

$$Upper\ frequency = 110\ Hz$$

Source: Industrial-Occupational Hygiene Calculations: A Professional Reference

63. Answer: A
Explanation: There are three general classes into which occupational noise exposures can be grouped: continuous noise, intermittent noise, and impact-type noise.

Continuous noise is normally defined as broadband noise of approximately constant level and spectrum to which an employee is exposed for a period of 8 hours per day, 40 hours per week. Exposure to intermittent noise can be defined as exposure to a given broadband sound-pressure level several times during a normal working day. The inspector or facility supervisor who periodically makes trips from a relatively quiet office into noisy production areas may be subject to this type of noise. Impact-type noise is a sharp burst of sound, and sophisticated instrumentation is necessary to determine the peak levels for this type of noise. Noise types other than steady ones are commonly encountered. In general, sounds repeated more than once per second can be considered as steady. Impulsive or impact noise, such as that made by hammer blows or explosions, is generally less than one-half second in duration and does not repeat more often than once per second. *Source: Fundamentals of Industrial Hygiene*

64. Answer: C
Explanation: Audiometric test should be pure tone, air conduction with test frequencies including as a minimum 500, 1000, 2000, 3000, 4000, and 6000 Hz (8000 Hz is also recommended). Noise-induced hearing loss is most prominent at the 3000-6000 Hz range. Speech and hearing sensitivity is best around 500-3000 Hz. *Source: Industrial Hygiene Reference and Study Guide, 3rd edition*

65. Answer: C

Explanation: The total for 90, 95, and 101 dB is approximately 102 dB. Eliminating 90 and 95 dB still leaves 101 dB in the room. Eliminating 95 dB still leaves 101 dB. Eliminating 101 dB leaves 90 and 95 dB which produces 96 dB. Eliminating 90 dB leaves 102 dB in the room. *Source: Noise and Hearing Conservation Manual, 4th Edition*

66. Answer: C

Explanation: Conductive soles minimize the likelihood of static charge build up and discharge. This protection is used in environments with combustible powder and vapors to reduce ignition sources.

Protective footwear requirements are referenced in the Department of Labor's Code of Federal Regulations (CFR) Title 29. General PPE requirements are given in the Occupational Safety and Health Administration's (OSHA's) standard 1910.132, and Foot Protection requirements are in 1910.136.

Per 29 CFR 1910.136(a), *"Each affected employee shall wear protective footwear when working in areas where there is a danger of foot injuries due to falling or rolling objects, or objects piercing the sole, and where such employee's feet are exposed to electrical hazards."*
29 CFR 1910.136 incorporates by reference the ASTM F2412-05 Standard Test Methods for Foot Protection, F2413-05 Standard Specification for Performance Requirements for Protective Footwear and the American National Standards Institute (ANSI) American National Standard for Personal Protection - Protective Footwear (ANSI Z41-1999 and Z41-1991).

On March 1, 2005, the ANSI Z41 reference was withdrawn and replaced by the ASTM Standards. ASTM F2412-11(Standard Test Methods for Foot Protection) and ASTM F 2413-11 (Standard Specification for Performance Requirements for Protective (Safety) Toe Cap Footwear are the most current footwear consensus standards

67. Answer: D

Explanation: Assigned protection factors are set in OSHA's respiratory protection standard 29 CFR 1910.134. See the table below for the assigned protection factors for each type of respirator.

Type of Respirator	Half Mask	Full Face Piece
Air-purifying respirator (APR)	10	50
Powered air-purifying respirator (PAPR)	50	1,000

Source: CFR 1910.134; osha.gov

68. Answer: C

Explanation: 1910.134(f)(1): The employer should ensure that employees using a tight-fitting face piece respirator are fit tested prior to initial use of the respirator whenever a different respirator face piece (size, style, model or make) is used, and at least annually thereafter. *Source: osha.gov*

69. Answer: D

    Explanation: Administrative controls that reduce employee exposures by scheduling reduced work times and worker rotation in contaminant areas. Employee training that includes hazard recognition and specific work practices that help reduce exposure is also valid. *Source: Fundamentals of Industrial Hygiene, 2nd Edition*

70. Answer: B

    Explanation: Wear time is the percent of time the respirator is worn during the time it is required. It is used to determine the effective protection factor.

$$wear\ time = \frac{time\ worn}{time\ required}$$

$$wear\ time = \frac{358}{360}$$

$$wear\ time = 99\%$$

Source: The Occupational Environment, Its Evaluation, Control, and Management, 3rd edition

71. Answer: A

    Explanation: The US Occupational Safety and Health Administration (OSHA) defines an APF as the workplace level of respiratory protection that a respirator or class of respirators is expected to provide to employees when the employer implements a continuing, effective respirator protection program as specified in its respiratory protection standard. *Source: The Occupational Environment: Its Evaluation, Control, and Management, 3rd Edition*

72. Answer: C

    Explanation: Scintillation is a class of radiation detection based on the energy transmission from radiation to a substance that responds to this energy transfer by emitting light. Photoelectric effect is the process of a gamma photon ejecting an electron and transferring most of the energy to the electron. The Compton effect is the process of a gamma photon ejecting an electron and a reduced energy photon, which may cause additional ionization. In pair production, the gamma photon enters the vicinity of a nucleus without striking it, thus causing an electron and positron to be created. *Source: Industrial Hygiene Reference and Study Guide, 3rd edition*

73. Answer: C

    Explanation: Progeny is the modern term for decay products. Historically, the term "daughters" was commonly used.

74. Answer: A
Explanation:

Step 1: Locate the QF factor for Alpha particles: 20

Step 2: Solve for REM

$$rem = rad \times QF$$

$$rem = 0.15 \text{ mrad/hour} \times 20 \text{ mrem/mrad} \times 7 \text{ hours}$$

$$= 21 \text{ mrem or } 0.021 \text{ rem}$$

Source: Useful Equations: Practical Applications of OH & S Math, 3rd Edition

75. Answer: D
Explanation: The EPA estimates 5,000-20,000 cases of lung cancer per year are related to inhalation of Radon. If Radon decays while inhaled, progeny are produced, all of which emit high-energy alpha radiation that causes lung damage.

76. Answer: B

$$X = 3.32 \ log\left(\frac{I_1}{I_2}\right)(HVL)$$

X is the shield thickness
I_1 is the incident intensity
I_2 is the exit intensity
HVL is the half-value layer

Step 1: Solve for X

$$X = 3.32 log\left(\frac{100 \ millirem/hour}{2 \ millirem/hour}\right)(0.0043 \ cm)$$

$$X = 0.024 \ cm$$

77. Answer: A
Explanation: An annular impactor head collects alpha, beta, and gamma emitting contaminants. An annular kinetic impactor head collects large airborne particles. The device does not collect radon and thoron. The approximate efficiency is 95%. *Source: energy.gov*

78. Answer: B
Explanation: For a frame of reference, consider that the innate human aversion response time to bright light, including invisible laser light, is approximately 0.25 seconds. Note that the aversion response does not occur with exposure to invisible radiation such as UV and IR. With this in mind, if a laser emits radiation for a time greater than or equal to 0.25 seconds, then it is defined as a continuous-wave (CW) laser. *Source: The Occupational Environment: Its Evaluation, Control and Management 3rd Edition, Volume 2*

79. Answer: D

Explanation: Damage mechanisms may be photomechanical, thermal or photochemical. Photomechanical effects, sometimes called photoacoustic effects, occur when brief pulses are incident on tissues. Such pulses may be generated by Q-switched or mode-locked lasers. Photomechanical effects (also called photoacoustic effects) can destroy tissues directly and may cause hemorrhaging, with blood collecting in the vitreous. Thermal effects affect the eye or skin, and occur in exposure times from microseconds to seconds. Thermal effects involve absorption of radiant energy by a chromophore (absorbing structure) such as melanin or hemoglobin. *Source: The Occupational Environment: Its Evaluation, Control and Management 3rd Edition, Volume 2*

80. Answer: B

Explanation: Elastosis or skin aging, melanoma (skin cancer), rash and reddening are chronic effects. Shock and burns are associated with ELF exposure. *Source: Applications and Computational Elements of Industrial Hygiene, Stern and Mansdorf.*

81. Answer: A

Explanation: UV-B and UV-C are primarily absorbed in the tissue of the cornea and conjunctiva. Corneal transmission ranges from 60% to 83% in the UV-A band, with much of the energy absorbed by the lens. Photokeratitis and photoconjunctivitis result from acute, high-intensity exposure to UV-B and UV-C. Commonly referred to as "arc eye" or "welder's flash" by workers, this injury results from exposure of the unprotected eye to a welding arc
or other artificial sources rich in UV-B and UV-C. Sunlight exposure produces these sequelae only in environments where highly reflective materials are present, such as "snow blindness" or sand. *Source: The Occupational Environment: Its Evaluation, Control, and Management 3rd Edition Vol. 2*

82. Answer: B

Explanation: Key characteristics of light sources are efficiency, color rendering index, and color temperature.
Efficiency –The ability of converting energy to visible light.
Color Rendering Index – A relative scale that rates how perceived colors of objects illuminated by a given source matches the color produced by the same object when illuminated by a reference standard light source.
Color Temperature – The color of a blackbody radiator at a given temperature. *Source: The Occupational Environment: Its Evaluation, Control, and Management 3rd Edition Volume 2*

83. Answer: D

Explanation: Commercially available welding curtains may be made of materials that are either opaque or transparent to visible wavelengths. Opaque materials include canvas duck, asbestos substitutes, and polymer laminates. Transparent welding curtains may allow visual contact with welders, reduce arc glare, and increase general illumination levels. *Source: The Occupational Environment: Its Evaluation, Control, and Management 3rd Edition Volume 2*

84. Answer: D

Explanation: Conduction is the transfer of heat between two objects from the hotter to the colder object. Convection is the transfer of heat by air movement. Radiant heat is the transfer of heat using electromagnetic radiation such as molten metal or the sun making the skin warm. *Source: Applications and Computational Elements of Industrial Hygiene, Stern and Mansdorf*

85. Answer: C

Explanation: Prickly heat is characterized by red papules in areas where clothing contacts skin and may be caused as excess sweat is absorbed by the keratinous layer of the skin. *Source: Applications and Computational Elements of Industrial Hygiene, Stern and Mansdorf*

86. Answer: A
Explanation:

Table: Heat Illness- Signs and Symptoms and First Aid Treatment

Heat Illness	First Aid Treatment	Signs and Symptoms
Heat Cramps	Salted fluids by mouth, or IV infusion	Painful spasms of muscles used during work. Onset during or after work hours.
Heat Exhaustion	Remove to cooler environment, rest in a reclined position, administer fluids. Rest until rehydrated.	Fatigue, nausea, headache, giddiness. Skin clammy and pale.
Heat Stroke	Immediate and rapid cooling by immersion in chilled water with massage or by wrapping in wet sheet with vigorous fanning. Medical attention needed.	Hot, dry skin Rectal temperature above 40.5°C Confusion, loss of consciousness, convulsions.

87. Answer: D
Explanation:

Heat Stroke – Occurs when the body's temperature regulation fails and body temperature rises to critical levels. Heat stroke typically results in loss of consciousness. Heat stroke requires immediate medical treatment.

Heat Exhaustion – Occurs when the body sweats profusely and has a rapid pulse. Signs and symptoms are headache, nausea, weakness, and thirst.

Heat Cramps – Muscle cramps caused by loss of salt and water through sweating. Heat cramps can be controlled by adequate consumption of fluids and salts. *Source: The Occupational Environment, its Evaluation, Control, and Management (S.R. DiNardi, Editor), American Industrial Hygiene Association*

88. Answer: A
   Explanation: Calculate the WBGT value

$$WBGT = 0.7 + 0.2GT + 0.1DB$$

$$WBGT = 0.7 \times 26 + 0.2 \times 35 + 0.1 \times 30$$

$$WBGT = 28° \, C$$

Since the employee is working outside for his entire shift, solar load (Dry Bulb Temperature) must be utilized. *Source: The Occupational Environment, its Evaluation, Control, and Management (S.R. DiNardi, Editor), American Industrial Hygiene Association*

89. Answer: D
   Explanation: The potential for exposure through the skin's mucous membrane is identified by the skin notation.

90. Answer: A
   Explanation: The skin consists of approximately 2 square meters of surface area and approximately 15% of body mass.

91. Answer: C
   Explanation: All but formaldehyde have been associated with decreased sperm count.

92. Answer: B
   Explanation: The concentration of a chemical in the body is dependent upon the amount absorbed. As a general rule, the longer a person is exposed and the higher the concentration, the greater the amount absorbed.

93. Answer: C
   Explanation: The key is occupational. In addition, dermatitis is specific: relating to the skin.

94. Answer: A
   Explanation: Aluminum is a relatively soft metal associated with shaver's disease or carborundum smelters lung.

95. Answer: B
   Explanation: There are four major classes of metal-working fluids widely available: straight oil, soluble oil, semisynthetic, and synthetic. Many metalworking fluids, except the straight oils, are mixed with water for use. Each has additives such as surfactants, biocides, extreme pressure agents, anti-oxidants, and corrosion inhibitors to improve performance and increase fluid life (refer to Appendix 2 for a listing of typical additives).

Straight Oil: This type of metalworking fluid is made up mostly of mineral (petroleum) or vegetable oils. Petroleum oils used for these fluids tend to be "severely solvent refined" or "severely hydrotreated" (refining processes that reduce cancer-causing substances called polynuclear aromatic hydrocarbons [PAHs] present in crude oil). Other oils of animal, marine, or synthetic origin can also be used singly or in combination with straight oils to increase the wetting action and lubricity. Straight oils can be recognized by an oily appearance and viscous feel. These materials may contain chlorinated and sulfur additives. This product is not diluted with water before use. Straight-oil metalworking fluids are generally used for processes that require lubrication rather than cooling. They perform best when used at slow cut speeds, high metal-to-metal contact, or with older machines made specifically for use with straight oils. Straight-oil MWF systems may require fire protection.

Soluble Oil: Soluble oil is also called emulsifiable oil. It is composed of 30% to 85% of severely refined lubricant base oil and emulsifiers to help disperse the oil in water. The fluid concentrate usually includes other additives to improve performance and lengthen the life of the fluid. Soluble oil products are supplied as concentrates that are diluted with water to obtain the working fluid. They may have colorants added. Soluble oils in general provide good lubrication and are better at cooling than straight oils. Drawbacks in using soluble oils, however, are that they sometimes have poor corrosion control, are sometimes "dirty" (i.e., machine tool surfaces and nearby areas become covered with oil or difficult-to-remove product residues), may smoke (they may not cool as well as semisynthetics and synthetics), and may have poor mix stability or short sump life.

Semi-synthetic: This type of metalworking fluid contains a lower amount of severely refined base oil, for example, 5-30% in the concentrate. Semi-synthetics offer good lubrication, good heat reduction, good rust control, have longer sump life, and are cleaner than soluble oils. They are comprised of many of the same ingredients as soluble oils and contain a more complex emulsifier package.

Synthetic: These metalworking fluid formulations do not contain any petroleum oil. They contain detergent-like components to help "wet" the part and other additives to improve performance. Like the other classes of water-miscible fluids, synthetics are designed to be diluted with water. *Source: OSHA Metal Working Fluid Manual*

96. Answer: A
   Explanation: *Phosgene* is created by the photo-oxidation and thermal decomposition of chlorinated hydrocarbons, which is possible in this scenario due to plasma cutting in a building that uses chlorinated solvents.

   Ozone has an odor that is described a reminiscent of chlorine with a slight metallic scent. It would be present during plasma cutting.

   Thermal decomposition of plasticizers would generally be associated with overheating (malfunctioning) equipment and the odor would be described as molten plastic. *Source: Patty's Toxicology, Vol 3, 5th edition*

97. Answer: A

Explanation: DCS is also called the "bends" and occurs when insufficient pressure is released from the body following exposure to increased pressure. It is more common in SCUBA divers but also occurs in caisson workers. Going from an area of high to low pressure allows nitrogen bubbles to form in the body, resulting in pain, narcosis, and even death. *Source: NIOSH-CDC Decompression Sickness*

98. Answer: B

Explanation: Mold remediation workers are one group of workers recognized as potentially having unacceptable exposures to mold. There are no federal health or safety standards or regulations specifically addressing exposures unique to mold remediation worker protection.

Fit-tested respirators with High Efficiency Particulate Air (HEPA) cartridges were originally required for any size job. The 2002 NYCDOH guidelines allow disposable respirators (N-95) as the minimum level of protection in work areas with up to 100 ft^2 of mold. Disposable coveralls and full-face respirators with HEPA cartridges continue to be recommended by NYCDOH for larger projects. *Source: AIHA, Assessment, Remediation, and Post-Remediation Verification of Mold in Buildings*

99. Answer: B

Explanation: Confined Space Standard 29 CFR 1910.146 defines a confined space as a space that is large enough and so configured that an employee can bodily enter and perform assigned work; has limited or restricted means for entry and exit; and is not designed for continuous employee occupancy. *Source: osha.gov, 29 CFR 1910.146*

100. Answer: A

Explanation: Numerous studies have found that workplace air and surface dust are the primary sources of occupational lead exposures. *Source: Patty's Toxicology Volume 2, 5th Edition*

Self-Assessment Exam 5

1. The gas or vapor is retained on the surface of a granular sorbent, physically and chemically unchanged. What method of extraction does this describe?

    A) Adsorption.
    B) Desorption.
    C) Absorption.
    D) Degradation.

2. It is accepted that airflow is proportional to the static pressure in the following manner:

$$\frac{Q_1}{\sqrt{SP_1}} = \frac{Q_2}{\sqrt{SP_2}}$$

    This formula can be applied in the following scenario: A Gemini® dual flow sample holder is being used with sample 1 calibrated to 0.05 L/m and sample 2 calibrated to 0.1 L/m both at a pressure of 5 inches WG. Assuming the actual pressure was 4 inches WG, what is the actual flow for sample 1?

    A) 0.06 L/m
    B) 0.055 L/m
    C) 0.04 L/m
    D) 0.045 L/m

3. Select the force or mechanism that is the basis for particle collection for an impactor.

    A) Diffusion.
    B) Inertia.
    C) Interception.
    D) Separation.

4. The theory of operation for a hand held PID is:

    A) UV light of specified energy ionizes a molecule creating a change in electrical current.
    B) Infrared light of specified wavelength ionizes a molecule creating a change in electrical current.
    C) Molecules are oxidized and the increase in heat is proportional to the concentration.
    D) Ionizing radiation splits the molecule and the resulting energy release is proportional to the concentration.

5. The sample flow rate for a pump was recorded as 1.7 l/m and a concentration of 100 mg/m^3 was determined based on the volume associated with the flow of 1.7 l/m. The flow rate was actually 2 l/m. What is the corrected concentration?

   A) 50 mg/m^3
   B) 85 mg/m^3
   C) 100 mg/m^3
   D) 117 mg/m^3

6. An industrial hygienist conducted an 8-hour TWA sampling for acetone, ethyl acetate, and ethyl ether. See concentrations below:

   Acetone: 500 ppm
   Ethyl Acetate: 100 ppm
   Ethyl Ether: 110 ppm

   Acetone's 8-hour TWA Permissible Exposure Limit (PEL) is 1,000 ppm. Ethyl Acetate's 8-hour TWA Permissible Exposure Limit (PEL) is 400 ppm. Ethyl Ether's 8-hour TWA Permissible Exposure Limit (PEL) is 400 ppm. What is the additive mixture exposure value for acetone, ethyl acetate, and ethyl ether, and does this value make the worker over exposed?

   A) 0.15, the worker is not overexposed.
   B) 0.88, the worker is not overexposed.
   C) 1.025, the worker is overexposed.
   D) 1.80, the worker is overexposed.

7. Quality control samples in a laboratory control which type of error?

   A) Systematic.
   B) Sample.
   C) Random.
   D) Pre-determined bias.

8. Given two spectrophotometer readings from two solutions, and the known equivalent molar concentrations, how is the molar concentration of an unknown solution determined from its spectrophotometer reading?

   A) Utilizing the principals of Fick's law.
   B) Utilize the principals of Boyles law.
   C) Utilize the principals of Bowes law.
   D) Utilize the principals of Beers law.

9. Which of the following is not true about the Beer-Lambert law?

    A) Relates the spectroscopic absorbance to the path-length of the sample cell.
    B) Uses the molar absorptivity as a constant of the proportionality.
    C) States the absorbance is inversely proportional to the analyte concentration.
    D) Correlates the observed spectroscopic absorbance of the concentration of the target analyte.

10. The most common method for analyzing metals is:

    A) Flame Ionization.
    B) Atomic Absorption.
    C) Electron Capture.
    D) Photoionization.

11. What does a thermal conductivity detector measure?

    A) Thermal conductivity of gasses.
    B) Thermal conductivity of liquids.
    C) Thermal conductivity of solids.
    D) All of the above.

12. Choose the statement that does not accurately describe High-performance Liquid Chromatography (HPLC).

    A) HPLC is a separation tool suitable for compounds that have high boiling points and low vapor pressures.
    B) HPLC Is commonly used for PAHs and have been derived for airborne organics, such as isocyanates and aldehydes.
    C) HPLC uses liquid as the carrier of mobile phase.
    D) All of the above accurately describe HPLC.

13. The thinnest skin (0.5mm) is located on the _____ and the thickest skin (3-4mm) is located on the _____.

    A) Wrist; Palm.
    B) Eye-lid; Elbow.
    C) Eye-lid; Palm.
    D) Wrist; Elbow.

14. What is the importance of breathing air through the nose?

    A) It breaks down all material that is on its way to the lungs.
    B) It moistens, filters, and warms the air that is on its way to the lungs.
    C) It moistens, filters, and cools the air that is on its way to the lungs.
    D) B & C.
    E) All of the above.

15. Choose the type(s) of photoreceptor cells located in the retina.

    A) Cone and dendritic.
    B) Dendritic and rod.
    C) Cone.
    D) Cone and rod.

16. What anatomical part of the ear is prone to the inflammation or infection otitis externa?

    A) Ear canal.
    B) Cochlea.
    C) Eustachian tube.
    D) Eardrum.

17. Which of the following terms describes a liquid in which a solute can be dissolved in?

    A) Vapor phase
    B) Solvent
    C) Solution
    D) Acid

18. Calculate the amount of liquid in mL (SG 83, MW 100) that must be vaporized in a 5 x 5 x 4 foot chamber to create a concentration of 100 ppm:

    A) 1.4 mL
    B) 1.9 mL
    C) 14 mL
    D) 19 mL

19. The killing or removing of all organisms from a surface is:

    A) Sterilization.
    B) Antisepsis.
    C) Disinfection.
    D) Decontamination.

20. Which class is the least dangerous in biosafety nomenclature?

    A) Class 4.
    B) Class 3.
    C) Class 5.
    D) Class 1.

21. Outdoor workers are potentially exposed to tick borne illnesses. Which of the following are illnesses that can be transmitted by a tick bite?

   A)   Byssinosis, Pneumoconiosis, Histoplasmosis.
   B)   Anaplasmosis, Ehrlichiosis, Lyme Disease.
   C)   Lyme disease, Histoplasmosis, Aspergillosis.
   D)   Influenza B, Hepatitis B, Lyme Disease.

22. Which of the following is a mold bulk sampling method?

   A)   Moisture meter and detection equipment.
   B)   Borescope testing.
   C)   Micro-vac dust collection.
   D)   Spore trap.

23. Giardia lamblia is an organism that lives in a host and causes adverse effects. Select the best description of this organism.

   A)   Toxin.
   B)   Parasite.
   C)   Fungi.
   D)   Arbovirus.

24. Choose the statement that best describes dry heat decontamination.

   A)   Sterilization of new, prepackaged medical devices (e.g., syringes and catheters) and in bulk package sterilization in the delivery of food industries.
   B)   Membrane filters are used to remove bacteria, yeast, and molds from biologic and pharmaceutical solutions.
   C)   Open flames and Bacti-Cinerators (tm) (an electrical device that dry-heats at 1600°F) are used to heat sterilize inoculation loops. Hot air ovens (160-180°C for 2 hours) are used for anhydrous materials (e.g., greases and powders). Incinerators are used to destroy infectious waste.
   D)   Boil (212°F for > 30 minutes) and pasteurization (161°F for 15 seconds, or 143°F for 30 minutes) kills vegetative cells but not bacterial spores. High temperatures cause denaturation of enzymes and kill organisms.

25.   A study was conducted among a group of employees at Company XYZ to evaluate exposure to acetone. The table represents eight Acetone exposure levels for each employee. The mean is 10.40 ppm.

Table: Acetone Exposure

Employee	Acetone Exposure (ppm)
1	15.9
2	20.6
3	11.9
4	4.1
5	2.5
6	7.5
7	12.3
8	8.4

Calculate the standard deviation.

A)   1.14 ppm
B)   2.70 ppm
C)   5.43 ppm
D)   6.03 ppm

26.   This use of the t-test is illustrated in a comparison of two analytical methods.

Suppose we have two methods being used to analyze for toluene. An atmosphere of toluene vapor in air is generated, and 10 samples are collected with method 1, and 10 samples are collected with method 2. The following results are obtained:

Method 1: mean = 75.51 ppm, SD = 3.15 ppm, n = 10
Method 2: mean = 74.23 ppm, SD = 2.98 ppm, n = 10

Perform the t-test and calculate the test statistic.

A)   0.40
B)   0.79
C)   0.93
D)   1.24

27.   What parameter is necessary for evaluating cumulative exposure?

A)   Arithmetic mean.
B)   Standard deviation.
C)   Geometric mean.
D)   Geometric standard deviation.

28. Choose the statement that best describes the Decision statistic.

    A) The distribution of a random variable with the property such that the logarithms of its values are normally distributed.
    B) An estimate of the parameter selected to represent the acceptability of an exposure profile.
    C) Parameters used to make estimates about the exposure distribution and underlying population.
    D) A quantity that describes a statistical population (e.g., mean and standard deviation, geometric mean, geometric standard deviation).

29. Choose the study design that identifies a group of workers with a disease and examines their past work history for potential exposures.

    A) Cross-sectional study.
    B) Case-control retrospective study.
    C) Case-control prospective study.
    D) Mortality study.

30. What type of bias fails to take into account other variables that are associated with both the disease and the exposure?

    A) Selection bias.
    B) Observational bias.
    C) Confounding bias.
    D) Information bias.

31. The Clean Air Act identifies two types of ambient air quality standards. One of these is to provide public health protection, including protection for the health of sensitive individuals, while the other is to provide public welfare protection, including protection against decreased visibility and damage to animals, crops, vegetation, and buildings. The two standards are:

    A) Mandatory, voluntary.
    B) Criteria, non-criteria.
    C) Human health, environmental health.
    D) Primary, secondary.

32. A "lapse rate" is the decrease in _____ with an increase in _____.

    A) Temperature; Elevation.
    B) Elevation; Temperature.
    C) Time; Temperature.
    D) Temperature; Time.

33. Control equipment is vital when dealing with pollutants. Four factors need to be identified when understanding if an air cleaner is needed. Three of the four factors are toxicity of the material, amount of material, and value of material. What is the fourth factor?

    A) Mass of Material.
    B) Carcinogenicity of Material.
    C) Government Regulations.
    D) Local Regulations.

34. The diagram illustrates what type of plume?

    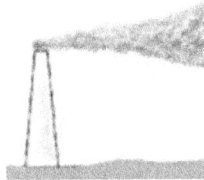

    A) Fanning.
    B) Fumigating.
    C) Looping.
    D) Coning.

35. Which of the following is not a good choice for particulate removal from an exhaust stream?

    A) Cyclone.
    B) Bag house.
    C) Electrostatic precipitator.
    D) Carbon capture and storage.

36. Fan material selection can be a factor when fans are operating at air temperatures substantially above or below 70°F. For fans with aluminum wheels, what is the maximum allowable operating temperature?

    A) 100°F
    B) 200°F
    C) 300°F
    D) No Temperature Restriction

37. A laboratory space requires six air changes per hour (6 ACH) to ensure a safe environment for the laboratory occupants. During a safety audit of the lab it was discovered that the laboratory ventilation was only delivering 4 ACH. The laboratory dimensions are 9 feet X 12 feet X 22 feet. Calculate the additional CFM of air that must be supplied to the laboratory space to achieve 6 ACH.

   A) 80 CFM
   B) 158 CFM
   C) 238 CFM
   D) 2,376 CFM

38. What is the friction loss in 20 feet of 10-inch diameter round stainless steel duct based on a velocity of 2000 FPM and nomograph values of K = 2.4 per 100 ft. and a VP of 0.25 in WG? Literature states the correction factor is 0.9.

   A) 0.12 inches WG
   B) 0.09 inches WG
   C) 0.11 inches WG
   D) 0.2 inches WG

39. A manometer on the suction side of a fan is reading 0.59 inches WG velocity pressure and 1.3 inches WG static pressure. What is the total pressure on the suction side of the fan?

   A) 0.47 inches WG
   B) 0.71 inches WG
   C) -0.47 inches WG
   D) -0.71 inches WG

40. Workers are handling solvents on a work surface approximately 10 inches from an unflanged exhaust hood that is 30 inches long and 2 inches wide. The target capture velocity is 80 FPM. The flow into the hood is 800 CFM. Calculate the capture velocity, and does the calculated value meet the target velocity requirement?

   A) 800 FPM, yes
   B) 1920 FPM, yes
   C) 67 FPM, no
   D) 104 FPM, yes

41. Select the correct pressure relationships for upstream of the fan:

   A) Total pressure +, static pressure -, velocity pressure +
   B) Total pressure -, static pressure -, velocity pressure -
   C) Total pressure -, static pressure -, velocity pressure +
   D) Total pressure +, static pressure +, velocity pressure –

42. What is hood entry coefficient for a hood with air flow velocity pressure of 1.4 inches WG and a hood static pressure of -1.9 inches WG?

   A) -0.23
   B) 0.11
   C) 0.86
   D) 2.60

43. Which of the following is not a disorder of the upper extremities?

   A) Epicondylitis.
   B) Carpal tunnel syndrome.
   C) Chondromalacia.
   D) Adhesive capsulitis.

44. Which of the following is not a work-related risk factor for musculoskeletal disorders?

   A) Repetition.
   B) Distribution.
   C) Force.
   D) Posture.

45. Carpal tunnel syndrome is:

   A) A respiratory disease resulting from breathing polluted air in tunnels where carbon monoxide is present.
   B) A problem in the wrist resulting from compression of the median nerve.
   C) A common illness of coal miners in the Carpathian Mountains.
   D) An elongation of the finger extensor tendons.

46. The application of ergonomics emphasizes:

   A) Selecting and training individuals to fit different jobs.
   B) Designing jobs and tasks to fit people.
   C) Decreasing worker complaint.
   D) Meeting OSHA standards.

47. What is the appropriate method when sampling for the aromatic hydrocarbon Styrene?

   A) OSHA 800.
   B) NIOSH 960.
   C) OSHA 1401.
   D) NIOSH 1501.

48.   When conducting sampling for lead, what is the recommended media?

 A) Solid Sorbent tube.
 B) 1 μm PTFE filter.
 C) .8 μm cellulose ester membrane filter.
 D) Silica Gel Tube.

49.   Control banding (CB) is a qualitative and semi-quantitative approach to risk assessment and management. A chemical is assigned to a band based on its:

 A) Hazard classification.
 B) Amount in use.
 C) Volatility/dustiness.
 D) All of the above.

50.   What do the letters ACGIH represent?

 A) American Center of Governmental Industrial Hygienist.
 B) American Conference of Governmental Industrial Hygienists.
 C) American Center of Governance in Industrial Health.
 D) American Conference of Governance in Industrial Health.

51.   Threshold Limit Values (TLVs) are expressed in which unit(s)?

 A) g and deciliters

 B) $\frac{mg}{m^3}$

 C) ppm

 D) $\frac{mg}{m^3}$ and ppm

52.   When testing for arsenic elemental and soluble inorganic compounds using the Biological Exposure Indices (BEIs), when should you conduct sampling for the determinant?

 A) End of a shift.
 B) End of the workweek.
 C) End of shift at the end of the workweek.
 D) Not critical.

53. Historical exposure monitoring has identified the top 3 chemical exposures at a manufacturing facility. The mean exposure is used as an indicator of routine exposure. Which of the three chemicals presents the most risk to workers based on the following information?

Chemical	Exposure Limit	Mean Exposure
Acetone	50 ppm	250 ppm
Benzyl Acetate	01 ppm	10 ppm
Ethyl Benzene	4.5 ppm	20 ppm

A) Acetone.
B) Benzyl Acetate.
C) Ethyl Benzene.
D) The risk is equal for all.

54. According to McGregor, Theory Y directs a people-centered approach. Which of the following is not a basic assumption of Theory Y?

A) Work is not a normal part of life.
B) People can exercise self-control and do not require threats to work effectively.
C) People commit to objectives based on their perception of rewards.
D) People seek responsibility.

55. When is it acceptable practice for a consulting industrial hygienist to provide sampling results directly to the worker who was evaluated?

A) If the employee asks for the results.
B) If the testing is being performed on Friday and the report must be sent before the end of the week.
C) It is not acceptable to provide results directly to the worker.
D) If the worker faces an immediate serious hazard related to the exposure.

56. The 5 S process is designed to ensure that improvements in the workplace are clearly visible, readily understood and consistently followed. Select the 5 S elements.

A) Sort, Set in Order, Shine, Standardize, Sustain.
B) Select, Sort, Store, Standardize, Sustain.
C) Sort, Systemize, Shine, Standardize, Sustain.
D) Sort, Shine, Segregate, Standardize, Sustain.

57. What process makes it possible to identify uncertainty and unpredictability of personal injury, property loss, business interruption, and liability?

   A) Fixed control management.
   B) Loss prevention management.
   C) Risk management.
   D) Prevention control management.

58. Out of the following techniques listed below, which is most likely to result in a positive safety record at a company?

   A) Utilize and implement a safety tool that will evaluate facility safety.
   B) Conduct safety meetings only after major incidents have occurred.
   C) Employ a CIH as the company safety director.
   D) Ensure supervisors and managers are accountable for safety with a cost accounting system for safety.

59. Which of the following correctly describes the JIHEEC?

   A) The JIHEEC publishes case studies of ethical dilemmas in numerous peer reviewed journals.
   B) The JIHEEC is an enforcement group or resolution board.
   C) The JIHEEC's mission is to promote an awareness and understanding of the enforceable code of ethics published by the ABIH.
   D) JIHEEC's acronym is Joint Industrial Hygiene Ethics Evaluation Committee.

60. What is the frequency of sound generated by a 12-bladed fan operating at 160 RPM?

   A) 32 Hz
   B) 54 Hz
   C) 71 kHz
   D) 9.9 kHz

61. What is the sound power level for a measured intensity of 10-3 W/m^2 where the reference intensity is 10-12 W/m^2?

   A) 30 dB
   B) 60 dB
   C) 90 dB
   D) 120 dB

62. Company XYZ is planning on adding additional ventilation to an enclosed paint booth. The new ventilation system is composed of two exhaust hoods. These hoods should ensure employees are not overexposed to the hydrocarbons in the paint. The hoods would be situated in the corner of the room and operate at 70 db. Two other hoods are also in the room and operate at 80 dB. What would the expected noise level be in the paint booth if the new ventilation system is installed?

   A)   70 dB
   B)   75 dB
   C)   83 dB
   D)   92 dB

63. There are two common types of sound waves. What are they?

   A)   Transverse and Inverse.
   B)   Longitudinal and Inverse.
   C)   Transverse and Longitudinal.
   D)   Longitudinal and Latitudinal.

64. What are the five areas of the hearing conservation program?

   A)   Exposure evaluation, engineering control, health screening, employee training, and audiometric exams.
   B)   Exposure evaluation, engineering control, administrative control, employee training, and audiometric exams.
   C)   Exposure evaluation, engineering control, administrative control, hearing protection, employee training, and audiometric exams.
   D)   Exposure evaluation, engineering control, hearing protection, employee training, and audiometric exams.

65. Select the definition of sound level:

   A)   The arithmetic average of the decibels measured over a period.
   B)   A combination of time-function variables.
   C)   The allowable dose obtained via integrated measurements.
   D)   Ten times the logarithm of the ratio of sound pressure squared, normalized with respect to reference pressure squared.

66. Personal protective equipment must be provided, used, and maintained in this condition "wherever it is necessary by reason of hazards capable of causing injury or impairment…"

   A)   Not previously worn.
   B)   In sanitary and reliable state.
   C)   Free from chemical contact.
   D)   Only by the person to who it was issued.

67. What is an acceptable non-engineering control utilized to minimize radiation exposure?

    A) Reducing time, increasing distance, and shielding in radiation exposure areas.
    B) Train employees to become aware of radiation exposure.
    C) Rotate employees to lower radiation exposure for each employee.
    D) Terminate employees exceeding radiation exposure limits.

68. ANSI Z88.2-1992 assigned a protection factor of _____ for a demand full-face self-contained breathing apparatus (SCBA). **NOTE**: Z88.2 was revised in 2015, and the assigned protection factors are aligned with OSHA in the revision.

    A) 10
    B) 100
    C) 1,000
    D) 10,000

69. A quantitative fit test is performed to determine whether a specific model and size of face piece fits an individual's face. Select an advantage associated with quantitative fit testing over qualitative fit testing.

    A) Utilizes specialized probes or adaptors.
    B) Requires training to operate.
    C) Purchase price.
    D) Real time documentation of fit.

70. Which of the following statements regarding breakthrough warning times is false?

    A) The reliance on warning properties to determine when breakthrough has occurred is no longer allowed under OSHA regulations.
    B) Warning properties to determine when breakthrough has occurred is useful for a change of schedule if the material has adequate warning properties.
    C) Breakthrough warning times are best calculated at the lab where the chemical is being used on a daily basis.
    D) None of the above.

71. This radiation causes direct ionization and has a range of approximately 2 cm in air because it is a highly charged particle. The charge makes it a serious internal hazard.

    A) X-ray.
    B) Alpha.
    C) Beta.
    D) Gamma.

72. Energies of atomic events may be stated in terms of electron volts, which is the kinetic energy imparted to an electron accelerated through an electrical potential of one volt. The energy of the gamma source Cesium 137 is approximately 0.67 MeV. How many electron volts is 0.67 MeV?

    A)   0.00067
    B)   0.067
    C)   6700
    D)   670000

73. In the radiation protection field, there is an assumption that even small doses have some chance of causing cancer. Therefore, it is important to do more than meet the regulatory limits. This concept is:

    A)   As low as realistically achievable.
    B)   Assume low and risk avoidance.
    C)   As low as reasonably achievable.
    D)   As low as realistically acceptable.

74. The US Nuclear Regulatory Commission established a TEDE of 5 rem (0.05 Sv). What is TEDE?

    A)   Transient Exposure Defined Energy.
    B)   Temporary Emergency Dose Equivalent.
    C)   Total Effective Dose Equivalent.
    D)   Total Emergency Dose Energy.

75. How many half value layers of shielding material are necessary to reduce exposure levels due to ionizing radiation source from 500 mrem/hour to 1 mrem/hour?

    A)   3
    B)   6
    C)   9
    D)   12

76. Which of the following answers is a critical organ for radioactive noble gases?

    A)   Skin.
    B)   Bladder.
    C)   Thyroid.
    D)   Lung.

77. Pulsed lasers can be set to which of the following modes of operation?

    A)   Normal pulse, Q-switched & Mode-locked.
    B)   High pulse, Q-switched & Mode-locked.
    C)   Low pulse, R-switched & Mode-unlocked.
    D)   Normal pulse, R-switched & Mode-unlocked.

78. Photochemical effects involving visible light up to 550nm target what anatomical part?

    A) Retina.
    B) Cornea.
    C) Pupil.
    D) Optic Nerve.

79. When exposed to UV radiation, the target organs are the skin, eyes, and immune system. Skin effects from occupational exposures include which of the following?

    A) Erythema, aging and cancer.
    B) Photosensitivity, aging and conjunctivitis.
    C) Erythema, photosensitivity, aging, and cancer.
    D) Photosensitivity, cancer and conjunctivitis.

80. Work lighting is necessary to provide visibility of work tasks and objects and to ensure safe working conditions. Illumination is the amount of quality of light falling on a surface. What are the general categories of lighting uses in a work environment?

    A) Ambient and task.
    B) Angle and accent.
    C) Task, angle and accent.
    D) Ambient, task and accent.

81. Optical density (OD or D1) is the quantity used to specify the ability of protective eyewear to attenuate optical radiation. The optical density equation is D1 = log10(ML/EL). What does the variable "ML" represent?

    A) Molecular level.
    B) Measured light.
    C) Measured (Calculated) level.
    D) Mean (Average) level.

82. A furnace operator, in a foundry, reports vision problems, and presents with red skin on the face and throat. Upon examination by the site nurse, retinal scarring is discovered. What is a likely cause of the injury?

    A) Microwave exposure.
    B) Pesticide exposure.
    C) UV exposure.
    D) IR exposure.

83. Which of the following is a heat conserving mechanism?

    A) Perspiration.
    B) Shivering.
    C) Cutaneous vasodilation.
    D) Vascular dysphoria.

84. A worker is working the night shift on the loading docks in Miami, Florida. The safety technician measures the Natural Wet Bulb = 85°F and the globe temperature = 84°F. What is the WBGT reading?

   A)   84.7
   B)   87
   C)   169
   D)   91

85. What is the work-rest regimen of a worker performing moderate work, and the WBGT reading is 29.4°C?

   A)   Continuous.
   B)   75% work, 25% rest.
   C)   50% work, 50% rest.
   D)   25% work, 75% rest.

86. Which of the following is an effective way to manage heat stress exposure for workers?

   A)   Schedule the most strenuous jobs early in the day to avoid the hottest part of the day.
   B)   Reduce the distance between the worker and radiant heat source.
   C)   Increase employee rest times when temperature increases.
   D)   All of the above.

87. An employee on a worker rotation is exposed to different work conditions throughout their shift. Assuming the employee is exposed to 32°C for 2 hours, 29°C for 2 hours and 25°C for 4 hours, what is the employee's average WBGT exposure during the shift?

   A)   90°F
   B)   95°F
   C)   82°F
   D)   78°F

88. The common target organ system for airborne organic solvent exposure is:

   A)   Lymphatic.
   B)   Hematopoietic.
   C)   Central Nervous.
   D)   Digestive.

89. The most common adverse health effect associated with occupational exposure to epoxy resins is:

   A)   Contact dermatitis.
   B)   Coughing and bronchospasm.
   C)   Dementia.
   D)   Esophageal burns.

90. What is considered the upper limit diameter of a particle that will reach the alveolar region of the lung?

   A) 15 um
   B) 0.5 um
   C) 5 um
   D) 50 um

91. Which of the following is not true about Shaver's Disease?

   A) Granulomas of the lung.
   B) Associated with aluminum industry.
   C) Typically not fatal.
   D) Associated with animal protein exposure.

92. The presence of methemoglobin in the blood is most likely associated with exposure to which of the following?

   A) Dimethylurea.
   B) Carbon dioxide.
   C) m-dinitrobenzene.
   D) Carbon monoxide

93. Sulfuric, nitric, and hydrofluoric acid can damage skin within moments. These compounds are best described as:

   A) Alkalines.
   B) Sensitizers.
   C) Atopic agents.
   D) Primary irritants.

94. Which task in the ferrous foundries is associated with the greatest risk of crystalline silica exposure?

   A) Mold shaping.
   B) Melting metal.
   C) Pouring metal into mold.
   D) Removing the cooled casting from the mold.

95. The following are useful approaches in building, design, construction, and operation for reducing the potential of mold amplification within the building.

   A) Installing UV lights at each building entry.
   B) Designing the HVAC system with the fresh air system fixed at 30% outdoor air.
   C) C.) Installing high efficiency filters on the HVAC system.
   D) Maintaining ambient temperatures below 65° F.

96. Which of the following would not be produced by plasma arc welding?

    A) Ozone.
    B) UV light.
    C) Infrared radiation.
    D) Metal dusts.

97. A respirator equipped with a regulator that is constantly flowing to maintain a pressure that is always greater than atmospheric pressure is a _____ respirator, which _____.

    A) Pressure demand, is the most protective type.
    B) Positive pressure, is likely to require a greater amount of air than other types.
    C) Negative pressure, will leak into the mask.
    D) Full face, has a higher assigned protection factor than a half face.

98. Which of the following is not a source of arsenic exposure?

    A) Pigment production.
    B) Insecticides and fungicides.
    C) Semiconductor manufacturing.
    D) Tire manufacturing.

99. Which of the following is a significant physical hazard to a worker performing abrasive blasting with steel shot?
    A) Noise produced by the high-velocity discharge from the nozzle and shot impact.
    B) Metal alloys of the abrasive blaster.
    C) Removal of coating material produced by the abrasive blaster.
    D) Heat generated from the abrasive blaster.

100. Immediately following an incident investigation, the investigator prints the digital pictures taken at the scene and makes notes on the pictures describing the context, orientation of the photographer, lighting, date, time and other information that may be helpful later in the investigation. What does this process describe?
    A) Chain of custody procedures.
    B) Spoiled evidence protocols.
    C) Forensic quality procedures.

1. Answer: A

   Explanation: Integrated air sampling involves the extraction of a gas or vapor from a sample airstream, followed by laboratory analysis. The two extraction techniques typically used include adsorption and absorption. *Source: Fundamentals of Industrial Hygiene 6th ed. NSC*

2. Answer: D

$$\frac{Q_1}{\sqrt{SP_1}} = \frac{Q_2}{\sqrt{SP_2}}$$

   Explanation:
   Insert the known values:

$$\frac{0.05 \; L/m}{\sqrt{5}} = \frac{Q_2}{\sqrt{4}}$$

   Rearrange and solve for Q_2:

$$Q_2 = \frac{0.05 \; x \; \sqrt{4}}{\sqrt{5}}$$
$$Q_2 = 0.045 \; L/m$$

3. Answer: B

Table: Particulate Sampling Techniques

Sampling Technique	Mechanism	Examples
Filters	A combination of inertial impaction, diffusion, interception, electrostatic attraction and forces of gravity.	Different types and sizes of fibrous membranes and nucleopore filters and their holders.
Impactors	Inertial impaction on a solid surface.	Cascade impactors- single and multi-jet, as well as single stage impactors.
Impingers	Inertial impingement/capture in a liquid.	Greenburg-Smith and midget impingers.
Elutriators	Gravity separation.	Horizontal and vertical.
Electrostatic Precipitation	Electrical charge and collection on an electrode of opposite polarity.	Two types, plate type and point-to-plane.
Cyclones	Inertia/centrifugal separation and collection on a secondary stage.	Tangential and axial cyclones of various sizes.
Thermal Precipitation	Thermophoresis- particles move under the influence of temperature toward decreasing temperatures.	Various devices, microscopic analysis

4. Answer: A

   Explanation: UV lamps (typically 10 eV, 10.6eV or 11.7eV) are used to ionize molecules in the gas stream. The ionized molecule bridges the gap between the anode and cathode generating an electrical current that is proportional to the concentration. *Source: The PID Handbook, Theory and Application of Direct Reading PID. Haag, W.*

5. Answer: B

   Explanation: Determine the ratio of the flow rates $1.7/2 = 0.85$, so 0.85 more air was drawn through the sample. Accordingly, the concentration 0.85 less than the original. 0.85×100 mg/m^3 = 85 mg/m^3.

6. Answer: C

   Explanation: Additive Mixture Formula

   $$\frac{C_1}{T_1} + \frac{C_2}{T_2} \cdots \frac{C_n}{T_n}$$

   $$\frac{500\ ppm}{1,000\ ppm} + \frac{100\ ppm}{400\ ppm} + \frac{110\ ppm}{400\ ppm} = .50 + .25 + .275 = 1.025$$

   Since the unity is greater than 1.0, the worker is overexposed due to the additive mixture effect.

   Source: TLVs and BEIs Based on Documentation of the Threshold Limit Values for Chemical Substances and Physical Agents & Biological Exposure Indices

7. Answer: A

   Explanation: The quality control samples address systematic error and include spiked samples and blanks. Systematic errors in experimental observations usually come from the measuring instruments. They may occur because there is something wrong with the instrument or its data handling system, or because the instrument is wrongly used by the experimenter. *Source: Topping, J. (1972). Errors of Observation and Their Treatment*

8. Answer: D

   Explanation: Absorbance *vs.* concentration is a linear relationship; therefore, use linear interpolation. Beers law Absorbance = $\log \frac{I_0}{I}$

9. Answer: C

   Explanation: The **absorbance is proportional** to the analyte concentration. Beer-Lambert relates the absorbance to the path length of the sample cell, uses molar absorptivity as a constant of the proportionality, Correlates the observed spectroscopic absorbance of the concentration of the target analyte and is useful for quantitative determination of the analyte concentration, but applies only to a restricted analyte concentration range. *Source: Rocky Mountain Center for Occupational and Environmental Health.*

10. Answer: B

    Explanation: Atomic absorption is an analytical technique that takes advantage of the characteristic absorption by metals of certain wavelengths of light. *Source: Applications and Computational Elements of Industrial Hygiene*

11. Answer: A

    Explanation: A thermal conductivity detector measures thermal conductivity of gasses. *Source: Applications and Computational Elements of Industrial Hygiene*

12. Answer: D

    Explanation: High Performance Liquid Chromatography (HPLC) can be used for the analysis of any organic compound that can be dissolved. The following characteristics describe HPLC. HPLC is a separation tool suitable for compounds that have high boiling points and low vapor pressures. HPLC is commonly used for PAHs and has been derived for airborne organics, such as isocyanates and aldehydes. HPLC uses liquid as the carrier of mobile phase. *Source: Applications and Computational Elements of Industrial Hygiene*

13. Answer: C

    Explanation: The thickness of the skin varies from 0.5 mm on the eye-lid (the dermis is thinnest here) to 3–4 mm on the palms of the hands and soles of the feet (the epidermis is thickest here). *Source: Fundamentals of Industrial Hygiene 5th Edition*

14. Answer: D

    Explanation: The nose serves not only as a passageway for air going to and from the lungs, but also as an air conditioner and as the sense organ for smell. The importance of breathing through the nose is obvious as it moistens, filters, and warms or cools the air that is on its way to the lungs. *Source: Fundamentals of Industrial Hygiene 5th Edition*

15. Answer: D

    Explanation: The retina, a thin membrane lining the rear of the eye, contains the light-sensitive cells. These photoreceptor cells are of two functionally discrete types: rods and cones. *Source: Fundamentals of Industrial Hygiene 5th Edition*

16. Answer: A

    Explanation: The ear canal is prone to the inflammation or infection (otitis externa) because of its high skin temperature and humidity. Bacterial and fungal infections occur more often under circumstances of heavy perspiration or head immersion. Common ear canal problems are swimmer's ear and dermatitis. *Source: Fundamentals of Industrial Hygiene 5th edition*

17. Answer: B

    Explanation: A solvent is a liquid in which a solid is dissolved to form a solution. *FIH 5th ed. National Safety Council*

18. Answer: A

    Explanation:

    Step 1: Calculate the volume of the chamber in Liters.

    $$\text{Volume} = 5 \times 5 \times 4 \text{ feet}$$

    $$\text{Volume} = 1000 \text{ ft}^3$$

    $$1000 \text{ ft}^3 \times 28.3 \text{ L/ft}^3 = 2830 \text{ ft}^3$$

    Step 2: Calculate the amount of liquid required for a target concentration of 100 ppm.

    $$2830 \text{ L} \times \frac{100\ L\ chemical}{1,000,000\ L\ container} \times \frac{1\ g-mole\ chemical}{24.45\ L} \times \frac{100\ g}{1\ g-mole} \times \frac{1\ mL}{0.83\ g}$$

    $$= 1.4 \text{ mL}$$

19. Answer: A

    Explanation: Sterilization destroys all microorganisms on the surface of an article or in a fluid to prevent disease transmission associated with the use of that item. *CDC Guideline for Disinfection and Sterilization in Healthcare Facilities.*

20. Answer: D

    Explanation: The CDC specifies 4 levels of containment, the lowest of which is Level 1 and the highest is level 4.

21. Answer: B

    Explanation:

    <u>Anaplasmosis</u>is caused by a bacterium called *Anaplasma phagocytophilum*, which leads to fever, chills, and headache within 1 to 2 weeks.

    <u>Ehrlichiosis</u> is caused by several species of the *Ehrlichia* bacteria, which leads to fever, chills, fatigue, and headache within 1 to 2 weeks.

    <u>Lyme Disease</u> is caused by the bacteria *Borreliaburgdorferi*, which leads to fever, headaches and joint aches within 3 to 30 days. If untreated, Lyme Disease can cause serious neurologic, cardiac, and joint problems.

    Although all of the choices are illnesses, only all of those in answer B are tick-borne illnesses. *Tick-borne Illnesses, Minimizing Risk to Outdoor Workers. Fred Kohanna, MD Professional Safety, June 2016*

22. Answer C

Explanation: According to the AIHA publication *Assessment, Remediation, and Post Remediation of Mold in Buildings*, a moisture meter is an assessment tool, borescopes are used for viewing inside wall cavities and other areas with restricted access, and a spore trap is used for air sampling. Other bulk methods include contact samples and wipe and surface-wash sampling.

23. Answer: B

Explanation: G. lamblia is a protozoan parasite that causes intestinal disorders. *Intermountain Healthcare Biohazard Lecture*

24. Answer: C

Explanation:
Table: Physical Agent Decontamination Techniques and Process/Application

Technique	Process/Application
Steam	Heat at 250°F under pressure (15-18 psi) in an autoclave. Most widely used and convenient method of sterilization.
Wet Heat	Boil (212°F for > 30 minutes) and pasteurization (161°F for 15 seconds, or 143°F for 30 minutes) kills vegetative cells but not bacterial spores. High temperatures cause denaturation of enzymes and kill organisms.
Dry Heat	Open flames and Bacti-Cinerators (tm) (an electrical device that dry-heats at 1600°F) are used to heat sterilize inoculation loops. Hot air ovens (160-180°C for 2 hours) are used for anhydrous materials (e.g., greases and powders). Incinerators are used to destroy infectious waste.
Ionizing Radiation	Sterilization of new, prepackaged medical devices (e.g., syringes and catheters) and in bulk package sterilization in the delivery of food industries.
Ultraviolet (UV) Radiation	Inactivation of viruses, mycoplasma, bacteria, and fungi. Least effective and least perfected method of sterilization. Not practical as a disinfectant of liquids.
Filtration	Membrane filters are used to remove bacteria, yeast, and molds from biologic and pharmaceutical solutions. Common spore sizes: 0.22μm, 0.45μm, and 0.8μm

25. Answer: D
   Explanation:

Table: Standard Deviation

Employee	Acetone Exposure (x_i)	$(\bar{x} - x_i)$	$(\bar{x} - x_i)^2$
1	15.9	-5.5	30.3
2	20.6	-10.2	104.0
3	11.9	-1.5	2.3
4	4.1	6.3	39.7
5	2.5	7.9	62.4
6	7.5	2.9	8.4
7	12.3	-1.9	3.6
8	8.4	2.0	4.0
Total	83.2	0	254.7

Calculate the standard deviation:

$$SD = \sqrt{\frac{(\bar{x} - x_i)^2}{n - 1}}$$

$$SD = \sqrt{\frac{(10.40 - x_i)^2}{8 - 1}}$$

$$SD = \sqrt{\frac{254.7}{7}}$$

$$SD = 6.03 \; ppm$$

If you are using the TI 30X IIS, use the following calculation keystrokes:

Step 1 – Set to STAT Mode using the second function of DATA key
Step 2 – Select 1-VAR and Enter key
Step 3 – Press DATA key

Step 4 – Enter Data (X_1, down arrow key, FRQ, down arrow key; X_2, down arrow key, FRQ, down arrow key; … X_n, down arrow key, FRQ, down arrow key)
Step 5 – Press the STATVAR key
Step 6 – Use arrow keys and select Sx
   Source: Industrial-Occupational Hygiene Calculations: A Professional Reference

26. Answer: C

Method 1: mean = 75.51 ppm, SD = 3.15 ppm, n = 10
Method 2: mean = 74.23 ppm, SD = 2.98 ppm, n = 10

Explanation:

Method 1: mean = 75.51 ppm, SD = 3.15 ppm, n = 10
Method 2: mean = 74.23 ppm, SD = 2.98 ppm, n = 10

Step 1: Calculate the SD_{pooled}

$$SD_{pooled} = \sqrt{\frac{(n_1 - 1)SD_1{}^2 + (n_2 - 1)SD_2{}^2}{n_1 + n_2 - 2}}$$

$$SD_{pooled} = \sqrt{\frac{(9)(3.15)^2 + (9)(2.98)^2}{18}}$$

$$SD_{pooled} = 3.07$$

Step 2: Calculate the test statistic

$$t = \frac{\bar{X}_1 - \bar{X}_2}{SD_{pooled}\sqrt{\frac{1}{n_1} + \frac{1}{n_2}}}$$

$$t = \frac{75.51 - 74.23}{3.07\sqrt{\frac{1}{10} + \frac{1}{10}}}$$

$$t = 0.93$$

The value of t in a table of the t distribution shows the probability associated with a value of t = 0.93 with 18 degrees of freedom (n-2) is >0.1. The interpretation is that we can conclude that the probability of the null hypothesis being correct is greater than 10%; therefore, we would not reject the hypothesis that the two sample means are equal. Put another way, we would not conclude that the two methods gave a different result. *Source: Industrial-Occupational Hygiene Calculations: A Professional Reference*

27. Answer: A

Explanation: A parameter is a quantity that describes a statistical population (e.g., mean and standard deviation, geometric mean, geometric standard deviation). The arithmetic mean is a measure of central tendency, calculated as the sum of all values in a population divided by the number of values in the population. The arithmetic mean is the correct parameter for evaluating cumulative exposure. *Source: A Strategy for Assessing and Managing Occupational Exposures 4th edition.*

28. Answer: B

    Explanation: Decision statistic - An estimate of the parameter selected to represent the acceptability of an exposure profile. For example, the 95th percentile is often used as the decision statistic when comparing an exposure profile to an OEL. *Source: Industrial-Occupational Hygiene Calculations: A Professional Reference*

29. Answer: B

    Explanation: Identify a group of workers with disease and examine their work history for potential exposures. The study period must start at a time when all of the participants were free of the outcome of interest and when first exposure can be ascertained. Most occupational epidemiology studies are retrospective because they seek to answer the question "Did exposure to agent "X" increase the risk for disease "Y." *Source: Epidemiology 5th Edition, Leon Gordis*

30. Answer: C

    Explanation: *Bias* is defined as any systematic error in the design, conduct or analysis of a study that results in a mistaken estimate of an exposure's effect on the risk of disease. *Selection bias* is the selection of individuals, groups or data for analysis in such a way that proper randomization is not achieved, thereby ensuring that the sample obtained is not representative of the population intended to be analyzed. *Observational bias* is gathering information on disease outcome obtained in noncomparable manner between exposed and nonexposed groups. *Confounding bias* is the failure to take into account other variables (i.e., smoking), which are associated with both the disease and the exposure. *Information bias* happens when the means for obtaining information about the subjects in the study are inadequate, so that as a result some of the information gathered regarding exposures and/or disease outcomes is incorrect. *Source: Epidemiology 5th Edition, Leon Gordis*

31. Answer: D

    Explanation: The Clean Air Act identifies two types of national ambient air quality standards. *Primary standards* provide public health protection, including protecting the health of "sensitive" populations such as asthmatics, children, and the elderly. *Secondary standards* provide public welfare protection, including protection against decreased visibility and damage to animals, crops, vegetation, and buildings. *Source: US EPA 2016*

32. Answer: A

    Explanation: A lapse rate is the decrease in temperature with an increase in elevation. The average value for the USA is 3.5°F/1000ft. = 6.5°C C/km. Note the sign; it is defined to be a positive number, indicating the temperature decreases as you go up in elevation. In an inversion, the lapse rate is negative, indicating that the temperature increases as you go up in elevation. *Source: Air Pollution Control Engineering, 2nd Edition*

33. Answer: C

    Explanation: Four factors are taken into account to figure out if an air cleaner is needed when controlling for pollutants: toxicity of the material, amount of material, value of material, and government regulations. *Source: Industrial Hygiene Reference and Study Guide, 3rd edition*

34. Answer: D

    Explanation: Coning plumes occur when there is a neutral or stable condition. *Source: Industrial Hygiene Reference and Study Guide. 3rd Edition*

35. Answer: D

    Explanation: Carbon capture and storage is the process of capturing waste carbon dioxide (CO_2) from large point sources, such as fossil fuel power plants, transporting it to a storage site, and depositing it where it will not enter the atmosphere, normally an underground geological formation. *Source: US EPA*

36. Answer: B

    Explanation: Fans with aluminum wheels have a maximum allowable temperature of 200°F. *Source: The New York Blower Company Engineering Letters, Letter 6, 1996*

37. Answer: A

    Explanation:

    $$\text{Room Volume} = 9 \text{ feet x } 12 \text{ feet x } 22 \text{ feet} = 2{,}376 \text{ ft}^3$$

    $$4\ ACH = 4\ ACH\ x\ 2{,}376\ ft.^3 = 9{,}504\ CFH\ or\ 158\ CFM$$

    $$6\ ACH = 6\ ACH\ x\ 2{,}376\ ft.^3 = 14{,}256\ CFH\ or\ 238\ CFM$$

    $$Additional\ CFM = 238 - 158 = 80\ CFM$$

38. Answer: C

    Explanation:

    Step 1: Calculate the loss

    $$SP_{loss} = \frac{K}{100\ ft}\ x\ VP\ x\ length\ ft\ x\ C_f$$

    Note: The k factor given in the nomograph was for galvanized metal, so use the stainless steel correction factor.

    $$SP_{loss} = \frac{2.4}{100\ ft}\ x\ 0.25\ x\ 20\ ft\ x\ 0.9$$

    $$SP_{loss} = 0.11 \text{ inches WG}$$

    Source: Laboratory Ventilation Workbook, Burton

39. Answer: D
   Explanation:

$$TP = VP + SP$$

VP = 0.59 inches WG
SP = -1.3 inches WG

Step 1: Solve for TP

$$TP = VP + SP$$

$$TP = 0.59 \; inches \; WG \; + (-1.3 \; inches \; WG)$$

$$TP = \; -0.71 \; inches \; WG$$

40. Answer: D
   Explanation:
   Step 1: Determine the hood type and formula to use for capture velocity

$$\text{The aspect ratio is } \frac{width}{length} = \frac{2 \; inches}{30 \; inches} = 0.067$$

By definition, if the aspect ratio is less than 0.2, then the hood is a slot hood. Therefore, this hood is an unflanged slot hood and according to ACGIH:

Q = 3.7 LVX

Note: L & X are expressed as feet and V as feet/minute

Step 2: Solve for V

$$800 \; CFM = 3.7 \; x \; \frac{30 \; inches}{12 \frac{inches}{foot}} \; x \; V \; x \; \frac{10 \; inches}{12 \frac{inches}{foot}}$$

$$800 \; CFM = 3.7 \; x \; 2.5 \; ft \; x \; V \; x \; 0.833 \; ft$$

$$\frac{800 \; CFM}{(3.7 \; x \; 2.5 \; ft \; x \; 0.833 \; ft)} = V$$

$$104 \; FPM = V$$

41. Answer: C
   Source: IH Workbook, 6th edition, Burton

42. Answer: C
   Explanation:

$$C_e = \sqrt{\frac{VP}{|SP_h|}}$$

$$VP = 1.4 \; inches \; WG$$
$$SP_h = -1.9 \; inches \; WG$$

Step 1: Solve for C_e

$$C_e = \sqrt{\frac{1.4 \; inches \; WG}{|-1.9 \; inches \; WG|}}$$

$$C_e = 0.86$$

Source: Industrial-Occupational Hygiene Calculations: A Professional Reference

43. Answer: C
   Explanation: Chondromalacia, also called chondromalacia patellae, refers to softening and breakdown of the articular cartilage of the kneecap. Epicondylitis is an elbow condition, carpal tunnel is associated with the wrist, and adhesive capsulitis is a shoulder condition. *Source: The Occupational Environment, Its Evaluation, Control, and Management. 3rd edition*

44. Answer: B

Source: The Occupational Environment, Its Evaluation, Control, and Management. 3rd edition

45. Answer: B
   Explanation: The result of compression of the median nerve in the carpal tunnel of the wrist. The tunnel is an opening under the carpal ligament on the palmar side of the carpal bones. Through the tunnel pass the median nerve, the finger flexor tendons and blood vessels. Swelling of the tendon sheaths reduces the size of the opening of the tunnel and pinches the median nerve and possibly blood vessels. The tunnel opening is also reduced if the wrist is flexed or extended or ulnarly or radially pivoted. *Source: Fundamentals of Industrial Hygiene 5th Edition*

46. Answer: B
   Explanation: Ergonomics is the study of human characteristics for the appropriate design of the living and work environment. Ergonomic researchers strive to learn about human characteristics (capabilities, limitations, motivations, and desires) so that this knowledge can be used to adapt a human-made environment to the people involved. This knowledge may affect complex technical systems or work tasks, equipment, and workstations, or the tools and utensils used at work, at home, or during leisure times. Hence, ergonomics is

human-centered, transdisciplinary, and application-oriented. *Source: Fundamentals of Industrial Hygiene 5ᵗʰ Edition*

47. Answer: D

   Explanation: According to the NIOSH Manual of Analytical Methods, the appropriate method when sampling for aromatic hydrocarbon Styrene is NIOSH 1501, the aromatic hydrocarbons method. The method specifies collection on a solid sorbent tube (coconut shell) and analysis done via gas chromatography-FID. The aromatic hydrocarbons use two different columns with Styrene designated for the group B column. *Source: NIOSH Manual of Analytical Methods 4ᵗʰ edition*

48. Answer: C

   Explanation: According to the NIOSH Manual of Analytical Methods, the recommended media when sampling for Lead is a 0.8 μm cellulose ester membrane filter. NIOSH 7082 and 7105 specify 0.8 μm MCE while NIOSH 7300 allows either the 0.8 μm MCE or a PVC filter. 7105 is a graphite furnace atomic absorption method that has a lower limit of detection (0.05 μg per sample). *Source: NIOSH Manual of Analytical Methods 4ᵗʰ edition*

49. Answer: D

   Explanation: Control banding (CB) is a qualitative and semi-quantitative approach to risk assessment and management. A chemical is assigned to a band based on its hazard classification, the amount in use, and its volatility or dustiness. This leads to one of the four, or a combination of the risk management approaches. The risk management approaches are summarized below.

   - General ventilation
   - Engineered controls, local exhaust ventilation (LEV) and/or partial enclosure
   - Containment with limited breaches
   - Special controls with expert input

   Source: The Occupational Environment: Its Evaluation, Control and Management 3ʳᵈ edition, Volume 1

50. Answer: B

   Explanation: The professional organization identified as ACGIH is the American Conference of Governmental Industrial Hygienists.

51. Answer: D

   Explanation: TLVs are expressed in ppm or $\frac{mg}{m^3}$. An inhaled chemical substance may exist as a gas, vapor, or aerosol.

   - A *gas* is a chemical substance whose molecules are moving freely within a space in which they are confined at normal temperature and pressure (NTP). Gases assume no shape or volume.
   - A *vapor* is the gaseous phase of a chemical substance that exists as a liquid or a solid at NTP. The amount of vapor given off by a chemical substance is expressed as the vapor pressure and is a function of temperature and pressure.
   - An *aerosol* is a suspension of solid particles or liquid droplets in a gaseous medium. Other terms used to describe an aerosol include dust, mist, fume, fog, fiber, smoke,

and smog. Aerosols may be characterized by their aerodynamic behavior and the site(s) of deposition in the human and the site(s) of deposition in the human respiratory tract.

TLVs for aerosols are usually established in terms of mass of the chemical substance in air by volume. These TLVs are expressed in $\frac{mg}{m^3}$.

TLVs for gases and vapors are established in terms of parts of vapor or gas per million parts of contaminated air by volume (ppm), but may also be expressed in $\frac{mg}{m^3}$. *Source: TLVs and BEIS Based on the Documentation of the Threshold Limit Values for Chemical Substances and Physical Agents & Biological Exposure Indices*

52. Answer: B

    Explanation: The test for arsenic is for the inorganic arsenic plus methylated metabolites in the urine to be conducted at the end of the workweek. Testing time and frequency are based on toxicological properties such as biological half-life and toxic effects. *Source: TLVs and BEIS Based on the Documentation of the Threshold Limit Values for Chemical Substances and Physical Agents & Biological Exposure Indices*

53. Answer: C

Chemical	Exposure Limit	Mean Exposure
Acetone	50 ppm	250 ppm
Benzyl Acetate	01 ppm	10 ppm
Ethyl Benzene	4.5 ppm	20 ppm

    Explanation: assuming no extraordinary health hazard exists for any of the chemicals, then a simple risk ratio may be used as part of a professional judgment decision. The risk ratio is $\frac{Exposure}{Exposure\ Limit}$.

    Accordingly, the risk ratios are: Acetone = 0.2, Benzyl Acetate = 0.1, and Ethyl Benzene = 0.225.

54. Answer: A

    Explanation: Theory Y states people view work as normal and do not dislike it, and most people can be innovative and tend to use a small portion of their intellectual potential. Theory Y workplaces tend to be participative in nature. *Source: The Occupational Environment: It's Evaluation, Control, and Management, 3rd Edition*

55. Answer: D

    Explanation: According the American Board of Industrial Hygiene Code of Ethics:
    A CIH or Candidates have a responsibility to:
    Maintain and respect the confidentiality of sensitive information obtained in the course of professional activities unless:

    - *The information is reasonably understood to pertain to unlawful activity*
    - *A court or governmental agency lawfully directs the release of the information*
    - *The client or employer expressly authorizes the release of specific information*

- *The failure to release such information would likely result in death or serious physical harm to the employee or the public*

56. Answer: A

    Explanation: The 5 S program focuses on visual order, organization, cleanliness and standardization. Many organizations add a 6th S – Safety. *Source: The Occupational Environment: It's Evaluation, Control, and Management, 3rd Edition*

57. Answer: C

    Explanation: The process of risk management is to identify the proper mix of loss control, risk retention, and risk transfer that the organization should use in dealing with its risk of personal injury, property loss, and liability.

58. Answer: D

    Explanation: The greatest impact on safety at any company is line management. In order to ensure a positive safety record, line management should be held accountable for their safety performance.

59. Answer: C

    Explanation: The mission of the Joint Industrial Hygiene Ethics Education Committee (JIHEEC) is to promote an awareness and understanding of the enforceable code of ethics published by the ABIH. JIHEEC is not an enforcement group or resolution board. JIHEEC publishes case studies of ethical dilemmas in the Synergist. *Source: American Industrial Hygiene Association*

60. Answer: A

    Explanation:

$$f = \frac{(N)(RPM)}{60}$$

$$N = 12$$
$$RPM = 160$$

Step 1: Calculate the Frequency

$$f = 12 \, x \, \frac{160}{60}$$

$$f = 32 \, Hz$$

Source: Industrial-Occupational Hygiene Calculations: A Professional Reference

61. Answer: C
    Explanation:

$$SPL = 10 \left(log \frac{I}{I_0} \right)$$

Step 1: Solve for L_i

$$SPL = 10 \, log \left(\frac{10^{-3}}{10^{-12}} \right)$$

$$SPL = 90 \, dB$$

Source: Occupational Safety Calculations: A Professional Reference, 2nd Edition

62. Answer: B
    Explanation:

$$SPL_f = 10 \, log \sum 10^{\frac{SPL}{10}}$$

Step 1: Solve for SPL_f

$$SPL_f = 10 \, log \, 10^{\frac{70}{10}} + 10^{\frac{70}{10}} + 10^{\frac{80}{10}} + 10^{\frac{80}{10}}$$

$$SPL_f = 83 \, dB$$

Occupational Safety Calculations: A Professional Reference, 2nd Edition

63. Answer: C
    Explanation: The two common types of sound waves are transverse waves and longitudinal waves. Transverse waves move horizontally and molecules move vertically. Longitudinal waves move vertically and molecules move horizontally. Sound waves are created by vibration. You can change their amplitude and frequency, but you cannot change the speed at which they travel through a medium. They are a constant that varies with temperature (i.e., the speed of sound for a given medium and temperature is constant). *Source: Industrial Hygiene Reference and Study Guide, 3rd edition*

64. Answer: D
    Explanation: The five areas of the hearing conservation program are exposure evaluation, engineering control, hearing protection, employee training, and audiometric exams. *Source: Industrial Hygiene Reference and Study Guide, 3rd edition*

65. Answer: D
    Explanation: Pressure squared is proportional to power. If subtracting the NRR from Dba, the 7-dB correction factor shall be used [dBA Exposure = Noise level dBA – (NRR – 7)]. This accounts for differences between A and C scales. *Source: Noise and Hearing Conservation Manual, 4th Edition*

66. Answer: B

Explanation: In addition to sanitary and reliable state, regulations and consensus standards require that PPE must be of safe design and construction, and that defective or damaged equipment must not be used. *Source: Industrial Hygiene Reference and Study Guide, 3rd edition*

67. Answer: A

Explanation: Minimizing radiation exposure shall be achieved by reducing time in exposure areas, as well as increasing distance from the source, and shielding from the radiation source. The aim of radiation exposures is to practice ALARA. As low as reasonably achievable (ALARA) goal is making every reasonable effort to maintain exposure to radiation as far below the dose limits as possible. *Source: nrc.gov; United States Nuclear Regulatory Commission*

68. Answer: B

Assigned Protection Factors ANSI Z88.2-1992

Type of Respirator	Half Mask	Full Face piece
Air Purifying	10	100
Atmosphere Supplying- SCBA (Demand)	10	100
Atmosphere Supplying- Airline (Demand)	10	100

ANSI Z88.2-1992

69. Answer: D

Explanation: Most models download the results of the fit test upon completion of the test. The results are direct and objective. The equipment is expensive and requires specialized adaptors for each model of respirator tested. Although operation is not complex, the operator must be trained and knowledgeable to obtain a good test. *Source: The Occupational Environment, Its Evaluation, Control, and Management, 3rd edition*

70. Answer: C

Explanation: The reliance on warning properties to determine when breakthrough has occurred is no longer allowed under OSHA regulations. Warning properties still provide a useful backup for a change schedule if the material has adequate warning properties. *Source: The Occupational Environment: Its Evaluation, Control, and Management, 3rd Edition*

71. Answer: B

Explanation: Alpha particles consist of two protons and two neutrons (Atomic Mass 4 – Atomic Number 2). Alpha particle radiation can be shielded by something as thin as a sheet of paper; however, it has a high energy and short range that can result in serious localized damage. Beta particles are high speed electrons with a charge of -1. They cause direct ionization but do not penetrate the skin deeply. Beta radiation does present a hazard to the lens of the eye. Neutrons are ejected from the nucleus with an Atomic Mass of 1 and no charge. They are highly penetrating, creating an internal hazard. *Source: The Occupational Environment: Its Evaluation, Control and Management, 3rd Edition.*

72. Answer: D

$$1 \text{ MeV (Mega-electron volt)} = 1,000,000 \text{ eV}$$

$$0.67 \ MeV x \frac{1000000 \ eV}{1 \ MeV}$$

$$= 670,000 \text{ eV}$$

Note: 1 meV (milli-electron volt) = 0.001 eV and 1 keV = 1000 Ev

Source: Useful Equations: Practical Applications of OH & S Math, 3rd Edition

73. Answer: C
Explanation: It is important to do more than meet the regulatory limits, since the majority of scientists accept the linear, no threshold hypothesis for radiation exposure. The concept of ALARA, as low as reasonably achievable, is followed. *Source: The Occupational Environment: Its Evaluation, Control and Management, 3rd Edition*

74. Answer: C
Explanation: The USNRC has a TEDE of 5 rem, Deep Dose Equivalent and Committed Dose Equivalent of 50 rem, Eye Dose Equivalent of 15 rem, and a Shallow Dose Equivalent to the Skin or Extremities of 50 rem.

75. Answer: C
Explanation:

$$I_2 = \frac{I_1}{2^{\frac{x}{HLV}}}$$

I_2 is the final exposure value
I_1 is the initial exposure value
x is the thickness of shielding material
HLV is the thickness of the material that equals one half-value layer

Note: $\frac{x}{HLV}$ determines the number of half value layers present, so for convenience, substitute a new variable: $Y = \frac{x}{HLV}$

Step 1: Solve for Y.

Note: When the unknown variable is in an exponent, take the log of both sides to mathematically bring the variable down "in front" of the log:

$$1 \ \frac{mrem}{hour} = \frac{500 \ \frac{mrem}{hour}}{2^Y}$$

$$2^Y = \frac{500 \frac{mrem}{hour}}{1 \frac{mrem}{hour}}$$

$$\log 2^Y = \log(500)$$

$$Y \log 2 = \log(500)$$

$$Y = \frac{\log(500)}{\log 2}$$

$$Y = 8.96578 \approx 9 \; half\,value\,layers$$

76. Answer: D

Explanation: A noble gas like radon is relatively insoluble, and after being inhaled, it is exhaled rather than being absorbed. If it decays during residence in the lung, a particulate daughter is produced. It is the progeny of radon, not radon per se, that contribute to lung dose. The daughter products exit as unattached ions, atoms, condensation nuclei, or attached to particles, all of which emit high-energy alpha radiation that causes lung damage. The target cell in the lung from radon exposure is the bronchial epithelium, which is the site of the majority of lung cancers considered to be caused by radon. *Source: The Occupational Environment: Its Evaluation, Control, and Management, 3rd Edition*

77. Answer: A

Explanation: The pulsed laser has a mode of operation which consists of the emission of either a single pulse or a series of laser pulses with pulse periods ranging from a few picoseconds to seconds. Pulsed lasers may be normal pulse, Q-switched, or mode-locked. *Source: The Occupational Environment: Its Evaluation, Control and Management 3rd Edition, Volume 2*

78. Answer: A

Explanation: Photochemical effects to the eye and skin primarily involve UV radiation, while retinal effects also involve visible light up to 550 nm (blue and green laser light). Photochemical damage is attributed to the photoproducts of light-induced chemical reactions or changes. *Source: The Occupational Environment: Its Evaluation, Control and Management 3rd Edition, Volume 2*

79. Answer: C

Explanation: The target organs for UV radiation are the skin, eyes, and the immune system. Skin effects that may be of importance from occupational exposures include erythema, photosensitivity, aging, and cancer. Ocular effects are photokeratoconjunctivitis, cataracts, and retinal effects. The most common adverse response of the skin to UV is erythema or sunburn. The International Commission on Illumination (CIE) erythema reference action spectrum indicates that the skin is most sensitive (lowest effective doses) from 250 nm to 300 nm. *Source: The Occupational Environment: Its Evaluation, Control, and Management 3rd Edition Volume 2*

80. Answer: D

Explanation: In the work environment, lighting is necessary to provide for visibility of work tasks and objects and to ensure safe working conditions. Illumination is the amount of quality of light falling on a surface. The three general categories of lighting uses are ambient, task, and accent. The first two uses are of prime importance in the work environment. Finally, the use of appropriate illumination principals and designs, as well as maintenance of that equipment, affects health, morale, comfort, and productivity. *Source: The Occupational Environment: Its Evaluation, Control, and Management 3rd Edition Volume 2*

81. Answer: C

Explanation: D_1 is the level of attenuation necessary to reduce the measured (or calculated) level (ML) to the exposure limit (EL). *Source: The Occupational Environment: Its Evaluation, Control, and Management 3rd Edition Volume 2*

82. Answer: D

Explanation: Microwaves heat internally. UV is mostly absorbed by the cornea. IR penetrates the retina and can cause burns to the retinal tissue and skin. *Source: The Occupational Environment: Its Evaluation, Control and Management Volume 2, 3rd Edition*

83. Answer: B

Explanation: Perspiration and cutaneous vasodilation are heat-dissipating mechanisms. Shivering and cutaneous vasoconstriction are heat conserving mechanisms. *Source: Applications and Computational Elements of Industrial Hygiene, Stern and Mansdorf*

84. Answer: A

WBGT = 0.7NWB + 0.3GT for indoor or outdoor with no solar load
WBGT = 0.7 x 85 + 0.3 x 84
WBGT = 84.7°F

85. Answer: C

Explanation: The ACGIH TLV is designed to prevent heat illness in healthy, acclimatized workers. The table shows WBGT limits for work at light, moderate, and heavy workloads.

ACGIH Heat Stress Threshold Limit Values- WBGT Threshold Limit Values, °C

Work-Rest Regimen	Heavy Work	Moderate Work	Light Work
25% Work 75% Rest	30.0	31.1	32.2
50% Work 50% Rest	27.9	29.4	31.4
75% Work 25% Rest	27.9 25.9	29.4 28.0	30.6
Continuous	25.0	26.7	30.0

86. Answer: D

Explanation: All of the answers are effective ways to manage heat stress to the employee. Where possible, it is a good practice to limit work during the afternoon hours since they are generally the hottest period of the day. If the work must be completed during the hottest times of the day, then proper consideration should be given to work rest cycles. *Source: The Occupational Environment, its Evaluation, Control, and Management (S.R. DiNardi, Editor), American Industrial Hygiene Association*

87. Answer: C
   Explanation:
   Step 1: Determine WBGT Average Temperature

$$WBGT_{AVG} = \frac{WBGT_1 \times T_1 + WBGT_2 \times T_2 + WBGT_n \times T_n}{T_1 + T_2 + T_n}$$

$$WBGT_{AVG} = \frac{(32 \times 2) + (29 \times 2) + (25 \times 4)}{2 + 2 + 4}$$

$$WBGT_{AVG} = \frac{222}{8}$$

$$WBGT_{AVG} = 28°C$$

Step 2: Convert from Celsius to Fahrenheit

$$T_{°F} = T_{°C} \times \frac{9}{5} + 32$$

$$T_{°F} = \left(28 \times \frac{9}{5}\right) + 32$$

$$T_{°F} = 82°F$$

The employee is exposed to an average WBGT of 82°F. In this two-part question, it was critical to remember to convert from Celsius to Fahrenheit before answering. *Source: The Occupational Environment, its Evaluation, Control, and Management (S.R. DiNardi, Editor), American Industrial Hygiene Association*

88. Answer: C
   Explanation: Organic solvent exposure typically produces central nervous system depression similar to intoxication.

89. Answer: A
   Explanation: Dermatitis, inflammation, and reddening from skin contact are the most common effects.

90. Answer: C
   Explanation: Although 10 um is considered inhalable, 5 um is the upper limit for alveolar deposition.

91. Answer: D
   Explanation: Shaver's Disease is associated with inhalation of aluminum fumes and dusts.

92. Answer: C
    Explanation: m-dinitrotoluene exposure is associated with methemaglobin formation while carbon monoxide exposure is associated with carboxyhemoglobin.

93. Answer: D
    Explanation: Primary irritants cause dermatitis by direct action on skin at the site of contact.

94. Answer: D
    Explanation: The removal of the casting is called shake-out. The silica becomes dry and brittle during the cast. It also undergoes some phase transformation to cristobalite and tridymite. *Source: Foundry Health Hazards publication, NOHSC, Government of Australia; and University of Utah lecture*

95. Answer: C
    Explanation: A properly designed, installed, and maintained HVAC is an important step in reducing the potential for mold amplification. Effective filtration that is well maintained can reduce the intake and circulation of mold and mold spores in the building. Fresh air fixed at 30% and ambient temperatures below 65°F are likely to result in decreased comfort and increased cost to operate.

    When designing buildings, preventing moisture from entering the space is important. The following are additional elements to be considered:

    - Controlling ground water around and under the foundation
    - Controlling surface water accumulation
    - Minimizing the entry outdoor mold material (airborne) into the building HVAC
    - Minimizing open windows and doors to the outdoor environment
    - Inspecting and eliminate water accumulation in HVAC system
    - Maintaining RH between 30 and 60%
    - Utilizing insulation, temperature, and humidity control to minimize condensation

    Source: ACGIH Bioaerosols: Assessment and Control, AIHA Assessment, Remediation, and Post-Remediation Verification of Mold in Buildings

96. Answer: D
    Explanation: The metal would be generated as a fume, not a dust. *Source: Patty's Toxicology, Vol 3, 5th edition*

97. Answer: B
    Explanation: To maintain a positive pressure inside the mask regardless of demand requires the regulator to provide a constant flow of air, which may actually increase the amount of leaking. The increased leaking will then require more air to be supplied. Pressure demand regulators are more desirable because the mask is maintained at a positive pressure and additional air is supplied when the demand is created.

98. Answer: D

Table: Arsenic and Compounds

Physical Form	- Metallic arsenic is a steel-gray brittle metal. - Arsenic trichloride is an oily liquid. - Arsenic trioxide is a crystalline solid.
Uses/Sources	- In metallurgy for hardening copper, lead and alloys. - Pigment production. - In the manufacture of certain types of glass. - In insecticides, fungicides and rodent poisons. - As a by-product in the smelting of copper ores. - As a dopant material in semiconductor manufacturer.
Exposure	- Inhalation - Skin absorption - Ingestion
Toxicology	- Arsenic compounds are irritants of the skin, mucous membranes and eyes. - Arsenical dermatoses and epidermal carcinoma are reported risk of exposure to arsenic compounds, as are other forms of cancer.

99. Answer: A

Explanation: Noise produced by the high-velocity discharge from the nozzle is the most significant physical hazard, while metal and other particulates are considered chemical hazards. The noise from the abrasive blaster can exceed 110 dBA. *Source: OSHA fact sheet, CDC-NIOSH hazard assessment*

100. Answer: A

Explanation: In the book *Root Cause Analysis Handbook, An Effective Guide to Incident Investigation* chain of custody procedures for photographs start with the photographer fully documenting the context, source, and relevant information related to the photograph.